OUR AGING BRAIN:
Changing and Growing

OUR AGING BRAIN:
Changing and Growing

By Harold W. Nash

ONTAROLINA PUBLISHING COMPANY
BURLINGTON, NORTH CAROLINA

OUR AGING BRAIN:
Changing and Growing

By Harold W. Nash

Published in the United States by
Ontarolina Publishing Company
PO Box 3293, Burlington, NC 27215
(336) 227-0000

tor: Tim Nash

Production/Design: Jan Cheves, AGA Publishing

Diagrams © 1999: Virge Kask, Illustrator

Publication Date: July 1999

Copyright © 1999 by Harold W. Nash, Ed. D.

ISBN: 0-9666162-0-0

Library of Congress Catalog Card Number 98-92099   1999

Table of Contents

Acknowledgements

Dedication

It is my great pleasure to dedicate this book to my wife, Lorraine, who showed much patience, faith, and common sense as we shared this new experience. Further tribute goes to Tim, Cheri, Allison, Ian, Marty, Eydie, Ryan, and Jayson.

Acknowledgements

The author wishes to thank the following who have kindly given permission for use of copyright materials:

From *How And Why We Age* by Leonard Hayflick Copyright (c) 1994 by Cell Associates, Inc. Reprinted by permission of Ballantine Books, a Division of Random House Inc.

Copyright (c) 1996 by Herbert Benson, M.D. *Timeless Healing*. Scribner.

From: *BRAIN, MIND, AND BEHAVIOR 2/E* by Bloom and Lazerson (c) 1985, 1988 by Educational Broadcasting Corporation. Used with permission of W.H. Freeman and Company.

Introduction And Table Of Contents from *Stop Aging Now!* by Jean Carper. Copyright (c) 1995 by Jean Carper. Reprinted by permission of HarperCollins Publishers, Inc.

Colin Dexter. *Death Is Now My Neighbor*, 1996. Copyright (c) by Crown Publishers, Inc.

From *Human Aging*. Augustine DiGiovanna, Copyright (c) 1994. Reproduced with permission of McGraw-Hill Companies.

From *The Human Brain and Spinal Cord* by Lennart Heimer Copyright (c) 1994. Permission for usage by Springer-Verlag New York, Inc.

From *Hemispheric Assymetry* by Joseph Hellige Copyright (c) 1993 by the President and Fellows of Harvard College. Reprinted by permission of Harvard University Press.

In addition I wish to thank a number of other people for the valuable contributions to the publication of *Our Aging Brain: Changing and Growing*. For their typing skills; Donnie Thompson, Peggy Corbett, and Amy Teske. For their time, advice, and reading of the manuscript: Lorraine Nash, Margaret Dixon, Christine Walsh, Alvin Westcott, Janice Baucom, James Baucom, Mario Rabozzi, David Parisian, Augustine DiGiovanna, and Lennart Heimer. Virge Kask for her artistic skills and the cover and nine diagrams. Special mention is made of Tim Nash for his diligence, time and valuable editorial skills. Jan Cheves contributed greatly to the production and design of the book.

CHAPTER 1

Introduction

The study of our brain began for me while on sabbatical leave at the University of North Carolina at Chapel Hill during the 1982 Spring Semester. The purpose of the leave was to study children who were described as autistic and learning disabled. This study developed an excitement for more information about our human brain. What was our brain like? How come I took it for granted for so long? What will I find out? Will any brain information help me in my teaching? In my personal life? Will I be interested in the brain? How will I ever be able to remember all that I read and study about the brain? It all seemed so vast and unfathomable.

When I started learning about the brain, I had very little upon which to build, as my science and anatomy background was not strong. I underwent the process of gathering information and ideas about the brain from the perspective of a professional teacher educator, not a scientist. Thus, I was looking at the human brain in terms of learning, memory, and early childhood development.

As I let friends and colleagues know of my increasing interest in the brain, they began to give me news articles, references, statements from journals, ideas from television programs, and a variety of photographs. Soon there was enough for me to develop a rough organizational system.

By early 1986, it seemed to me that enough pertinent ideas and material were available for a professional education graduate course. *The Brain and Classroom Teaching* was presented during the 1987 Spring Semester to twenty-eight brave elementary and secondary education teachers. We all learned a great deal together. Since then, courses such as *Learning Styles / Teaching Styles*; *Your Child's Growing Mind*; *Care and Feeding of the Brain*; *Sex, Hemispheres, and Learning*; and *The Brain: Teaching and Learning* have been presented at Alamance (N.C.) County Community College, and at the State University of New York at Oswego.

My interests in the brain have moved initially from anatomy to neural transmission to the evolutionary development of the brain. Next came the study of embryonic development to hemispheric differences to gender differences to learning styles. I moved on to study more anatomy, then to brain diseases to neurotransmitters to hormones to myelination to MRI (magnetic resonance imaging) and CAT (computerized axial tomography) images to holding a human brain in my hands, and now to an interest in our aging brain. The interest in our aging brain was partially fueled by noticing subtle changes in my own brain behavior and that of age-mates. Some faces lost their names. What did we have for lunch? Some appointments were missed. Some changes were annoying and puzzling.

Questions that have stayed with me since the beginning of my study are: What is the evolutionary position of our brain today? How did our brain get to be the way it is today? What could teachers know about the brain that would be helpful to them in their everyday classroom management and teaching? What might people like to know about their brains? What is useful and helpful to know about the brain?

As new information about our brain began to appear in the media, more was included about our brain as it ages. The question that formed was what would be of interest about our aging brain to senior citizens and relatives of senior citizens? My decision was to provide information appropriate for persons ages forty-five and above, who are relatively uninformed about the brain and its use in today's culture and technological environment.

This book is organized in a way that will allow you to develop some understanding of our marvelous brain. Its chapters share a variety of ideas related to our brain message-sending, intricate timing of development, difficulties that may occur, and some thoughts about our aging process. "Keeping Your Brain Healthy" is the chapter where mostly good news is shared. It is the place where a variety of information, activities, strategies, recommendations and possibilities are listed which could assist us as we age and as we encourage our brains to change and grow. The three appendices — diagrams, vocabulary and responses to myths or misconceptions — should give you additional insights into our brain. Appendix IV provides you with the opportunity to obtain more brain information. The bibliography contains a list of books which I found extremely helpful in writing this book.

The information, diagrams, vocabulary, and concepts that are included in the book are those I found most exciting, reasonable and significant as I began my focus on the aging brain. My birthdate is April 11, 1930. There are places in this book where I could not resist including myself in the aging brain picture, so I did just that. My approach to the organization and sequence of information probably should be attributed to the sequential nature of my left hemisphere. I hope your right hemisphere will permit you to see the "big picture" as your two hemispheres join to allow you to enjoy your brain and this book.

Some of my thoughts and rationale need to be shared as they relate to the content of the book. As mentioned, the audience is people aged forty-five and older who are relatively uninformed about our brain. They are the main focus of this book. Since starting the book two of my main concerns were the amount of scientific information to include and how much or how little repetition of terms and concepts should be present.

Let me attempt to put those concerns into a larger picture: how people study the brain and then talk or write about what they see and know. Often a brain researcher/writer examines the brain from his own perspective: his interests, his priorities, his purposes, and his own state of knowledge of the brain. He places his new knowledge in and around what he already knows and into some framework with which he is already comfortable. He may adopt someone else's scheme of organizing knowledge and use that person's anatomic labels. Or instead he may find that someone else's labels and definitions get in the way of what he would like to find out. An individual may adopt his own scheme for seeing and labeling the brain. That individual may consider our brain from only his scheme and then may perceive another organizational scheme as some what deficient or inappropriate or incomplete. In addition, the brain itself defies easy, simple, and absolute labeling, defining, and knowing. Two examples may help. The brain cells are called neurons. Various sources mention that these neurons may range in number from one billion to one hundred billion. The same sources number the connections that one neuron may have with another neuron from one to one thousand. It is extremely difficult to count neurons and all their connecting fibers. The limbic system, a main location for our emotional life, fits this puzzle too. One source may list four brain parts as belonging to the limbic system. Another source may list six parts while a third source lists seven parts.

So what to include and how to describe it? Some scientific information is included for particular reasons. Other terms are used for other reasons. Some of the vocabulary is used to satisfy my own need to share information about the brain. Some vocabulary is used to satisfy the natural curiosity and interest of some readers. Also terms like genes, chromosomes, proteins, peptides, dopamine, serotonin, basal ganglia, hippocampus, myelin, and dendrites are all words I have read in newspaper and magazine articles in the recent past. I am quite certain these words and others will continue to appear often in articles and on television.

How much repetition should be present? Some readers have commented that they had noticed some repetition. Others said that the repetition helped them become more familiar and comfortable with the inherent ideas. They also reported that their understanding of the brain grew through the repetition of terms and concepts.

You may also notice slightly different percentages may be reported for apparently very similar situations, age groups or diseases. These data have been accumulated at different times from a variety of studies using somewhat different populations.

A word or two about the brain itself may be in order.

One of our difficulties is that we are using our own brain to study our brain. The brain is difficult to study and classify. Some of the brain information organizing schemes are quite arbitrary, but also helpful. Other times they may impede our understanding. In writing about the brain, it is awkward to try to be complete, accurate, consistent, precise, general, and selective all at the same time. One starts, moves forward, tries to maintain focus, seeks and receives advice, and then makes decisions. In the end, any errors, inaccuracies, should haves, could haves, and mistakes are the fault of the author. I accept full responsibility for any and all those deficiencies.

CHAPTER 2

Twenty-Five Myths or Misconceptions

The following items are to encourage you to think about our brain. Some of the statements are reminders of commonly held misconceptions about the brain; others are reflections of ideas which are very prevalent in the media today. Some items may be true, but may seem quite odd at the same time. Each of the statements is discussed at one time or another within the book. In case you do not notice the particular discussion, I will talk about each item in Appendix III. Please read each one now and think about our brain. I have placed a "T" (true) of "F" (false) at the end of each item.

1. A big head means a big brain. (F)
2. Eating a lot of fish will help your brain function be better. (T)
3. We only use about ten percent of our brain's total capacity. (T)
4. A person is either a "left brained" or a "right brained" person. (F)

5. The older we get, the poorer our brain operates. (F)

6. Smoking, alcohol and other drugs have no effect on our brain. (F)

7. Alzheimer's disease and multiple sclerosis are diseases only of elderly people. (F)

8. There is nothing a person can do to prevent strokes. They are just unlucky things. (F)

9. The brains of men and women age the same way at the same rate. (F)

10. The food we eat has nothing to do with a healthy brain. (F)

11. There is nothing we can do to counteract the forgetfulness we encounter as we age. We just accept it. (F)

12. Our brain has some parts to it that are older in evolutionary terms than other parts. (T)

13. Men have bigger brains than women and use them differently. (T)

14. Our brain cells begin to die soon after we are born. (T)

15. By age ninety, we probably have lost about twenty percent of the weight and size of our brain. (T)

16. We may have one whole hemisphere of our brain surgically removed, still live and our brain function is close to normal. (T)

17. Every minute, one-and-a-half pints of blood flow through the brain. (T)

18. We cannot be absolutely certain that a person has Alzheimer's disease until an autopsy is performed. (T)

19. Our brain uses about twenty percent of our body's total energy and nourishment needs. (T)
20. Our brains were originally designed for self-protection. (T)
21. Alzheimer's disease and Parkinson's disease patients usually die from the complications of their disease. (T)
22. The rate of progress of Alzheimer's disease is always the same regardless of the age of onset. (F)
23. Our brains seem to be somewhat at a loss to deal with the challenges of our modern day culture. (T)
24. Orange juice is very helpful for the revival or recovery of dying or dead brain cells. (F)
25. We are at the mercy of the brain developed from the genes of our parents. (F)

CHAPTER 3

Aging Definitions and Hypotheses

P rior to inspecting some of the major aging hypotheses, it is important to examine various definitions of human aging, including this author's point of view. The assumptions and hypotheses should then make more sense to the reader.

One of Leonard Hayflick's thoughts in his book *How And Why We Age* (1994), is that "Aging is not merely the passage of time. It is the manifestation of biological events that occur over a span of time." In that book, he explores many significant positions from which to view the aging process.

Jean Carper, in her 1995 book *Stop Aging Now*, says that "Aging — the detrimental changes that occur as you get older — is actually in large part a monumental, progressive deficiency disease." She describes in her book how we may combat particular deficiencies.

Richard Besdine is quoted in Kathy Keeton's 1992 book *Longevity*. He maintains that "Aging doesn't necessarily mean that you must be sick, senile, sexless, spent, or sedentary." Also in the same book, T. Franklin Williams believes that "In most ways, aging is a remarkably benign series of processes. People who lead responsible lifestyles and who are spared some of the common diseases of aging can be phenomenally healthy and active in their late years."

Robert E. Ricklefs and Caleb Finch in their *Aging: A Natural History* (1995) describe aging as "progressive changes during the adult years that often, but not always, reduce an individual's viability." Their text also examines patterns, theories, evolution and genes as those topics are related to the aging process.

In his book, *Human Aging, Biological Perspectives* (1994), Augustine G. DiGiovanna maintains that aging is better understood once we accept the notion that human "developmental changes are irreversible normal changes in a living organism that occur as time passes." He goes on to distinguish among chronological, cosmetic, social, biological, economic and psychological aging.

The literature and my own experiences have provided me with some beliefs about aging and the aging process. It seems to me that aging is a process during which all parts of our body change due to the influence of our environment, both internal and external, and to our genetic luck as well as unavoidable physical accidents. There are a variety of external environmental factors which definitely affect our life expectancy. Among these factors are health care, marital status, employment, level of education and income, air pollution, smoking, alcohol, toxic chemicals, and prevention of disease measures. Aging is a phenomenon which affects each of us differently, and we show those differences in highly individual fashions. Aging is something that happens to each of us, but not in exactly the same way to all of us. Major factors in our reaction to age-related changes are our ability to accept these changes and our willingness to deal with them. Our aging brain, if we give it a chance, can be very instrumental in helping us adjust to these changes. For example, we may devise ways to help us remember appointments or times for medication. Also our brain can help us make plans to allow for our slower reaction time when driving.

Given the assumption that aging is an integral part of life, it must be regarded as an eventual outcome of normal growth and development, rather than a mere decline. This belief is supported and accepted by many who write and study about aging.

It is important to realize that aging in a human is quite different from the process of aging in the animal world. Animals, it is believed, endure their aging situation because they are not capable of foreseeing it. Humans, on the other hand, know, see and sense that they are getting old. People understand that, to a certain extent, old age can be changed depending on how they prepare for it, how they perceive it, accept it, and how they will adjust to it.

Overriding the hypotheses about the aging of our brain is the notion that aging is natural and inevitable for every living creature. Also, a part of this thinking is that aging must be regarded as an eventual outcome of our human growth and development. Many hypotheses about why we age seem to be rooted in genetic mechanisms. Others are based on internal or external environmental influences.

A. According to one hypothesis, each person's genetic program contains specific "aging" genes, which are switched on at a certain time of life in the same fashion as genes initiating puberty.

B. Another hypothesis is that in later life the organism simply runs out of genetic information and then the biological changes of aging follow.

C. A third hypothesis states that the genetic program is subject to random damaging events over time and, therefore, essential proteins do not get produced. Instead, cells produce proteins which are inactive or are actually harmful.

D. Other theories implicate the immune system, suggesting that it reacts adversely to the proteins that are produced as a result of damage to the genetic program — that is, the body reacts to its own products as if they were foreign substances. It produces antibodies in an immune-system reaction, and increasing numbers of such immune reactions would produce the changes seen in aging. One such theory is called the free radical theory.

There are at least two other aging hypotheses which fit under the heading of non-genetic based theories — the cross linkage and the endocrine or hormone theories. The cross-linkage theories say particular molecules and certain chemicals become linked together and this bonding restricts the movement of materials and parts of the body, leading to malfunctioning and aging. One endocrine theory supposes that aging takes place when a particular hormone is released by the pituitary gland (an endocrine gland). This released hormone changes the functioning of cells enough so that a biological aging takes place. Some call this theory the "death hormone theory" since the changes produced by this hormone do result in eventual death. Researchers believe that the production of this hormone and the resulting process may be slowed by reducing the amount of food eaten.

The preceding hypotheses about aging should provide you with some understanding of how researchers and theorists view aging in the human body, and therefore perhaps these views are helpful when considering our aging brain. Examination and verification of these hypothesis may be occurring as we read, or may be taking place in various research sites around the world. Life in the future may actually be accomplished in different ways through biochemical and surgical manipulations and gene therapy. That "life," however, may be quite different from life as we know it today. Researchers and philosophers are struggling with serious ethical questions as they consider possible changes in our genetic code, neuron regeneration and transplants of various types.

CHAPTER 4

Important Concepts About The Brain

The notion of "important concepts about the brain" originated from my early study of the brain. Quite often, the same information came up again and again, and it seemed to be basic and necessary to developing a foundation for further understanding of our brain. Students studying the brain continued to ask many of the same questions early in their courses. This basic information and responses to students' questions evolved into fifteen important concepts. Perhaps others will be added as new information becomes available.

1) The 1990's were declared "The Decade of The Brain."

In November 1990, President George Bush, at the encouragement of many learned and research oriented organizations, declared the 90s as the <u>Decade of the Brain</u>. The purpose was to sponsor and to encourage more research by a wide variety of academic disciplines and to share the accumulation of brain information among those disciplines. The long range goal was the development of new syntheses and new perspectives about the brain.

2) Each brain is similar to every other brain.

Every person throughout the world has a brain that is similar in appearance, size, weight, anatomical parts, color, function, and other characteristics. There is no such thing as a particular ethnic brain (Irish, Italian, Brazilian, Australian, American, etc.). People in various parts of the earth may use their brains differently than others due to environment, culture, tasks, and personal needs.

3) Each brain is unique and therefore slightly different from every other brain.

There is a saying that there are as many different brains as there are faces. Each person's brain is affected by its embryonic development, its genetic heritage from both mother and father and their many ancestors, various levels of hormones, its neurotransmitters, injuries, nutrition, exercise, stress, and overall health.

4) Each brain is said to be the result of evolutionary and environmental changes since our earth was formed about 4,500 million years ago.

Among the factors involved are said to be changes in climate, inter-group mingling, cell health, luck, the Ice Ages, needs of animals and humans, survival of the species that led to humans as we know them today, and our ever-changing human culture.

5) Our brain size has not changed much in the last 35,000-45,000 years.

Our brain's overall size and weight is described as being on a growth plateau since the fairly quick disappearance of the Neanderthal population and the appearance of the Cro-Magnons. Theorists credit the lack of brain size change to the size of the birth canal and the fact that until quite recently our brain size and function seemed to have served us well in our ever changing culture. There are some now who believe that our world culture has been changing so rapidly since World War II, that it has presented our brain function and capacities with very serious challenges.

6) Each brain weighs about three pounds.

A healthy, normally functioning adult brain weighs about 1400 cc or about three pounds with the male brain being a bit larger and maybe heavier than the female brain due to the overall larger male body size.

7) Each part of our brain is connected to most other parts by neurons.

Each part of our brain is connected to and interacts with other brain parts by billions of neurons, through axons, dendrites, synapses, neurotransmitters, and other chemicals.

8) Our brain contains 10 billion to 100 billion neurons (brain cells).

These neurons contain axons of varying lengths and

dendrites to help make billions and maybe trillions of important message-sending connections.

9) Our brain's health depends on what we do and what we eat for necessary nourishment.

Both physical and mental activity along with significant groups of food are necessary for maintaining long term healthy brain functioning. Our brain's health also depends upon what we do not eat or drink or inhale (alcohol, nicotine, marijuana, cocaine, for example).

10) Our brain continues to grow or remodel itself throughout our life.

Until recently, conventional wisdom said that our billions of brain cells (neurons) begin to die shortly after our birth and continue to die throughout our life. Now that wisdom is being questioned. Recent research shows that active and challenging mental activities, and changing one's lifestyle may foster an increase in the number of new dendrites and synapses. Recent evidence states that our brain cells may not die as quickly as once thought, and in fact, may be capable of regeneration. Hopefully, time will provide further clarification of these notions.

11) There is usually no such thing as a complete left brain person or a complete right brain person.

We use both hemispheres. Some people tend to use one hemisphere more than the other, depending on the activity or tasks at hand. The corpus callosum allows the two

hemispheres to "talk to each other." A hemispherectomy —
which takes place because of damage to the removed hemisphere due to strong and numerous epileptic seizures —
may remove one complete hemisphere. This surgery could
therefore cause a "one-hemisphere" person.

12) Each hemisphere is contralateral as it controls most of the opposite side of our body.

Our eyes and ears are both contralateral and ipsilateral,
meaning the information we take in with our eyes and
ears is delivered to both hemispheres at the same time by
different routes.

13) Various parts of our brain seem to be responsible for particular tasks.

Research is beginning to show that responsibilities for
these activities are not as localized in particular sections
of our brain as was originally thought.

14) Our brain allows us to think about what we are, where we are, and who we are.

It helps us make sense out of our world as we are continually bombarded 24 hours a day with information. It
helps us select, prioritize, and decide. Sleep apparently
gives us a rest from this continual thinking and allows us
to process the information we have received.

15) Every day we are finding out more and more about our brain.

Newspapers, magazines, journals, television, books and
the world wide web continually update our perspectives

about our brain. As new information about gene therapy, fetal cells, neurosurgery, human growth factors, temperature change, brain cell regeneration, vitamins, brain disorders, research and the changing of old assumptions is presented to us, our view of our brain is always evolving.

CHAPTER 5

Typical Brain Functioning

The foundation for this chapter is from Richard Restak's 1994 book, *Receptors*, Chapter Two. It provides quite a clear, thoughtful, and comprehensive view of the magical function of our brain.

I have harvested many of his significant ideas, information and concepts from that chapter in order to describe how a healthy, normal brain functions day to day. It is hoped that by possessing some information about normal brain function, a better understanding of the changes in brain function due to the aging process will occur.

For the purpose of inspecting our brain more closely, we may examine it by using the anatomic labels which have been passed down to us through time. As we examine our brain and identify its separate parts by name, we must constantly remember that it functions as a dynamic whole. Each element functions in relation to every other part. The method for our examination is to begin at the outer surface and move inward toward its central part. We will concentrate on our emotions, our behavior and our memory as they are affected by our aging.

The outermost part, the cerebrum, is separated into the left hemisphere and the right hemisphere and is what we see in most drawings or photographs of the brain. Each hemisphere has certain information for which it has processing responsibilities. Each hemisphere generally is divided into four parts: the frontal, parietal, temporal, and occipital lobes (see diagrams 1 and 3). There is another lobe in each hemisphere that may be seen by pulling out the temporal lobe and looking behind it. This insula lobe has some connections to at least the amygdala, hypothalamus and the brain stem. It seems to be involved in at least our taste and smell. A brief, general description of each of the four lobes listed above may be helpful. At the front and top of our head, behind the forehead, are the largest lobes, the two frontal lobes. They allow us to think, to consider consequences of our behavior, to make plans for the future, to consider philosophical, ethical, religious and moral questions. These thoughtful activities, functioning through the frontal lobes, are among those elements which allow us humanness and set us apart from other mammals (see the vocabulary appendix for more information about the frontal, parietal, temporal and occipital lobes).

The two parietal lobes, along the top of the brain, help us process functions of our sensory cortex: for example, our sensations of touch and skin sensations. Also, near the sensory cortex is the motor cortex, located in the frontal lobes. The motor cortex helps process those movements we choose to make which are different from our reflexive actions.

The two temporal lobes are located on the sides of our brain. Among their responsibilities are language, hearing, some parts of our memory, and our sense of time and self.

The two occipital lobes, located at the back part of the brain, are responsible for processing our vision. These occipital lobes receive information from our eyes as it is transmitted back through the optic nerves then crosses over at the optic chiasm and finally proceeds to the visual cortex at the rear of our brain. This visual transmission occurs in various amounts of milli-seconds depending upon the task.

The various lobes of the brain are all involved in the production of speech, but not necessarily all at the same time. Often, areas of the lobes operate in conjunction with one another. For example, listening to words activates areas of the temporal lobes in both hemispheres. Speaking words activates areas in the temporal, parietal, and frontal lobes, as well as in the cerebellum and along the top center of the brain. The two hemispheres of our brain look very similar. Each controls the opposite side of the body, and each processes information in very different ways. Various pieces of literature characterize the left hemisphere as processing information in analytic fashion that is breaking it down into its particular parts while being specialized for language and logic. The right hemisphere is described as looking at language and information from a wholistic point of view — looking at the complete, big picture — and being specialized for visual spatial activities such as geometric figure identification and tasks involving form and distance. The left hemisphere is described as looking at the individual trees, while the right hemisphere looks at the whole forest.

The two hemispheres are connected by a collection of nerve fibers called the corpus callosum (see diagram 4). The corpus collosum allows the two hemispheres to "talk to each other" and helps the two hemispheres to act in conjunction as they help our brain carry out its many functions.

Just inside and below the two cerebral hemispheres is a collection of brain structures roughly organized in the shape of a ring — the limbic system. Generally, the limbic system consists of the amygdala, hippocampus, septum and basal ganglia. Some authors also include the pituitary gland and the hypothalamus. It is connected to almost every other part of the brain and spinal cord, which make up our central nervous system. The significance of the limbic system is its vital role and responsibility for our feeling and expressing of emotions. Actually, all emotions and feelings, like happiness and sadness, are processed in the limbic system. Also, the limbic system is the place where many recent advances in chemical brain management and manipulation occur. A variety of drugs and counseling techniques are available which may influence our emotional behavior in both positive and negative ways.

Near the limbic system are the thalamus and hypothalamus (see diagrams 2 and 4). These two components are located near the base of the brain and above the pituitary gland. The thalamus processes the impulses of each of the senses, except smell. The hypothalamus is just below the thalamus. It is about the size of a thumb tip and has the richest blood supply in our entire body. From this tiny structure arise feelings of pleasure, punishment, hunger, thirst, sexual arousal, aggression, fear and rage. Along with its connection to, and help from, the nearby pituitary gland, it regulates hormone levels, appetite, and body temperature. With its connection to our brainstem, the hypothalamus maintains our homeostasis, our body's internal equilibrium. Homeostasis is a vital cog in our total human survival. The hypothalamus helps us maintain a necessary and generally even body temperature of 98.6 degrees Fahrenheit.

Situated beneath the hypothalamus and thalamus are the pons and medulla, which are both located in the brain stem. The brain stem contains areas which monitor blood pressure, temperature, breathing and heart rate. The nerves responsible for these activities are called the autonomic nervous system, since they happen without our knowing about them. There are drugs available which can cause powerful, dangerous and even life-threatening changes in our minds and our brains since they affect our autonomic nervous system.

As human beings going through the process of aging, we are naturally concerned about those brain functions to which we have become accustomed — memory, imagination, language, perception and creativity. Some authors would also include altruism along with these other functions. A realization that should be fairly important to us is that our brain's elaborate structure and its billions of interconnections seem to have evolved to operate the marvelous body processes that keep us alive. Communication among the billions of neurons that make up the brain is a highly significant element in our complex and creative daily life. The neurons receive information from other neurons. Synapses consider the information and then send messages which affect every other organ and cell in our body.

The main functional unit of the brain is the neuron (see diagram 5). It is quite different from other cells in the body since its main task is to process information. The main sections of the neuron are the cell body, the axon, the dendrites, and the synapse. The cell body produces all the necessary proteins and chemical substances to allow for neuron functioning and existence. The nucleus of the cell body, exactly like the nuclei in all other cells, contains our entire genetic share of DNA (Deoxyribonucleic acid).

Another element of the neuron is the axon. It is a single tubular extension away from the cell body and is of varying lengths up to a yard long. It conducts brain messages away from the neuron cell body to the synapse. Myelin, an insulation-like wrapping around most axons, greatly assists the speed at which these brain messages flow along the axon to the axon terminal. At the axon terminal and at the synapse, with the help of various neurotransmitters, the messages are passed to the dendrites and cell bodies of other networks.

These dendrites appear similar to roots of trees. They are actually numerous branches of the cell body. They receive messages from other neurons and the environment. The dendrites contain receptor sites which are designed for receiving neurotransmitters, which help carry the brain messages to the neuron.

This message-communication system takes place across a tiny space — the synaptic gap. Peter Russell in his 1979 *The Brain Book* describes this gap as being one five-thousandth of a millimeter in width (see diagram 5 and 6). The terminal of the axon projects into this tiny narrow synaptic gap. Vesicles are located in the axon terminal. These vesicles store and release the neurotransmitters when it is appropriate for the continuation of the brain messages. This process is called neural transmission.

A very important and fascinating relationship between a neurotransmitter and its receptor was described in 1900 by Paul Ehrlich. He introduced the notion that a neurotransmitter is to its receptor as a key is to a lock. This simple description has increased in complexity as more and more research has taken place over the succeeding years. Generally, each neurotransmitter possesses a particular molecular structure which fits the particular molecular structure of the receptor site. At times there may be neurotransmitters, slightly different from one another, competing for a receptor site. However, it is believed that the receptor will only accept one neurotransmitter at a time.

Chapter Nine, Significant Neurotransmitters, identifies particular neurotransmitters which have significant roles in our brain function as we age. For now, we just want to mention that neurotransmitters can be either excitatory or inhibitory and may be described by four main chemical types. The first, and most prevalent, are simple amino acids. They are involved in "rapid point-to-point communications between neurons." They are found in our diet and we come by them naturally. Included here are glycine, glutamate, and aspartate.

The second type is a group called the catecholamines. Included here are epinephrine, norepinephrine and dopamine. The third type are called indolemines. Included in that group are serotonin and melatonin. The catecholamines and indolemines fit into a classification called the monoamines.

The fourth chemical type includes histamine, nitric oxide, and neuropeptides. These neuropeptides are molecules made up of short chains of amino acids. Included in these neuropeptides are the endorphins, Substance P, and Substance K.

All of the neurotransmitters influence information transfer and movement with our brain. Some facilitate message sending. Still others facilitate neural transmission in other neurotransmitters. These neurotransmitters are extremely important in sending brain messages from neuron to neuron and among neurons. Their presence or absence is one of the more important considerations in our aging brain function and our physical behavior.

Richard Restak (1994) says that "The chemical diversity provided by all these substances allows the brain cells to exhibit a great flexibility and subtlety of response. In fact, one of the most exciting discoveries in brain research in recent years has been the discovery that neurons may utilize several neurotransmitters rather than a single one. This suggests that each neuron is capable of a greater variation in response than was considered possible only a few years ago. It is now believed that this wide repertoire of responses at the molecular level forms the basis for the rich behavioral complexity of our lives."

Our brain is indeed responsible for the "rich behavioral

complexity of our lives." Its hundreds of billions of neurons send messages to thousands of other neurons. It may be impossible to imagine the total of all the cell-to-cell inter-communications. The neurotransmitters encourage, restrict, or modulate our brain messages as they function in our brain as it is affected by its own chemistry, electricity, and magnetic forces. When something disrupts this marvelous dynamic relationship of neurotransmitters, chemistry, electricity, timing, genes, gender, internal and external environment, and personal experiences, our brain function is affected, slightly to seriously. As we age, many of us experience a diminishing of the operational efficiency of many of these various anatomical parts, their relationships and the cerebral forces that therefore affect the typical brain function we come to know, expect, and accept as young adults.

CHAPTER 6

Neural Transmission

One of the most fascinating and most highly significant functions of our brain is the way our brain cells or neurons communicate among each other and therefore transmit messages all over the brain and at the most appropriate times. This message-sending system of our neurons is also one of our brain functions which is often affected as we move through our aging decades. The following six paragraphs are reprinted from Robert Sylwester's 1995 book, *A Celebration of Neurons.* Sylwester's information provides a brief explanation of neural transmission. One of the most exciting and necessary concepts of a basic understanding of our brain function is that of neural transmission.

Writes Sylwester, "Neuron cell bodies and their many dendrite extensions constantly receive various levels of excitatory and inhibitory information from related neurons (see diagrams 5 and 6). This information is averaged within the cell body at the axon hillock (located where the axon leaves the cell body). Think of the axon hillock as fulfilling the thermostat function for a neuron. In a house, for instance, a thermostat maintains a comfortable heat level in a room by monitoring the heat level in the room and sending a message to the furnace when warm air is needed. But the temperature in a room differs in different places — perhaps 98.6 degrees on someone's face, 60 degrees on the window pane, and 150 degrees on the surface of a coffee cup. Such a system is designed so that a thermostat defines and maintains the room's temperature at whatever the temperature is at the thermostat's location. The axon hillock's monitoring system, however, is designed to average the various levels of information received.

"If the average input at a given moment reaches the neuron's firing threshold, an action potential develops, and the message moves rapidly along the axon to the terminal. The movement of a neural message along an axon has been likened to an electrical charge. It does have some similarities, but neural messages don't move in the same way that electrical currents do. It is also more complicated biochemically than the following brief functional explanation.

"The inside of an axon has a slight negative charge and the fluids outside the axon have a slight positive charge," Sylwester continues. "When a neuron reaches its firing threshold, it propagates a signal down the axon that rapidly opens and closes a series of channels in the axon. When a set of channels opens, positively charged sodium ions from the fluids outside the neuron enter the axon. This action briefly changes the charge inside that part of the axon from negative to positive, and also triggers the opening of the next set of channels. The process is then repeated with the next set of channels. Think of a row of dominoes falling over. Each domino pushes the next one, just as each set of channels opens the next set.

"After a set of channels opens, the sodium ions are pumped out, the channels close, and that part of the axon once again has a negative charge-until the next action potential propagates down the axon.

"One type of glial cell wraps itself around long axons, creating a kind of insulating layer called myelin. This wrapping process reduces the number of functioning sodium channels along the axon, and so speeds up the message. Think of an unmyelinated axon as a slow local train (5 mph) that stops at every station and a myelinated axon as a fast express train (200 mph) that stops infrequently.

"When the axon's wave of permeability to sodium ions (the sequential opening and closing of channels) reaches the axon terminal, calcium ions enter the terminal, triggering the release of packets (vesicles) of neurotransmitters into the synapse, where they attach to the appropriate receptors on the dendrites and/or cell body of the postsynaptic neuron-and thereby pass their neuron's message to the next neuron."

In addition to Robert Sylwester's previous text on neural transmission, it is important to provide a bit more information about what happens as our brain helps us talk to ourselves and others. We begin by mentioning again the positive and negative ions and polarization.

There is a fluid that surrounds all the cells of the body. In this fluid, there are positive and negative ions which are distributed evenly and freely in equal amounts, and they neutralize each other's charges. The ions of sodium, potassium, calcium, and magnesium all have a positive charge. In contrast, the ions of chloride, phosphate (a combination of phosphorus and oxygen), and other complex acids, which are made by cells from carbon and oxygen all have a negative charge.

Inside the brain's neurons are most of the body's proteins. The proteins are most often in the form of ions having a negative charge. Because of this, the neuron is described as being negatively charged. Due to the relative absence of positively charged particles inside the brain cell, there is a fairly strong electrical force trying to pull the positively charged ions into the cell. However, there is a border crossing guard on duty. This guard is called the plasma membrane or external cell membrane. The plasma membrane surrounds the neuron and does not permit all the outside substances equal right of passage to the inside. When the neuron is resting, this negative charge is continued. A number of things need to occur in order for a neuron to be active and they all seem to happen almost simultaneously.

A combination of channels (open and closed), ion pumps, plasma membrane selectivity, voltage differences, excitatory neurotransmitters, inhibitory neurotransmitters, synaptic vesicles, action potential, receptor sites, reuptake, and depolarization all combine, cooperate, coordinate, and react to begin, continue, or limit a succession of action potentials down the axon. These marvelous, exquisitely timed processes ensure there is no loss of neural signal or message or impulse along the entire length of the axon.

Neurotransmitters carry out their various communicative and transmission functions at the synapse. A synapse is that very narrow gap which separates the axon terminal of a presynaptic neuron from the dendrites of another neuron (see diagram 6). The dendrites contain receptors. Again, think of the receptor as a lock and the neurotransmitters as a key. The shape of the transmitters (key) interacts and combines with the shape of the receptor (lock). If it is a good match, the neurotransmitter transmits or releases its message into the postsynaptic neuron at that particular receptor site.

A neurotransmitter sends either an excitatory or inhibitory message to the receiving neuron. An excitatory message helps to increase the subsequent communicative action of the postsynaptic neuron, and an inhibitory message helps to reduce the subsequent communicative actions. Think of an on/off switch, or in some situations, a light-dimmer switch. The chemical composition of the neurotransmitter interacting with its target receptor determines the nature, complexity, and strength of the message.

Neural activity in our brain is fortunately much more inhibitory than excitatory. At any moment, we focus our attention, limit our activity, and ignore most of our memories. Imagine, with a principally excitatory brain that continually attended to everything, carrying out all possible actions, and had continual open access to all prior experiences! What a terrific and actual headache that would be, all the time!

The aging process seems to affect the various elements of our neural transmission in a number of ways. Our neurons die steadily and most often are not replaced. Some existing neurons may be able to "take over" for missing ones. Levels of some neurotransmitters change as we age. Dopamine lessens in the case of Parkinson's disease. Myelin may begin to waste away. Shrinkage of brain tissue affects our hemispheres, particularly in the hippocampus. The initial "fine-tuning" that characterized our neural transmission system just may not be possible and our message sending and receiving may not be as it once was.

A very significant part of our neurotransmission is the role played by our neurotransmitters. A later chapter examines particular neurotransmitters more carefully.

CHAPTER 7

Changes in the Aging Brain

The phrase "senior moment" has been in our vocabulary recently. A relative used it to explain the situation in which we find ourselves when we go into the kitchen to get something but can't remember what. Also, when we begin to say something but then find we can't remember what we were going to say. Let's identify some possibilities for the existence of our "senior moments."

The overall structure and sequence of information in this chapter may be attributed to the 1976 *Atlas of the Body and Mind*, Claire Rayner, Editor. The sections on early middle years, middle years and old age have provided helpful guidelines.

In almost all cultures and societies, the time between ages thirty and forty-five is considered by many people to be among their best years. These years are considered to be the time when there is a "coming together" of an individual's personal, public and family life. During this period, we tend to reach the height of our physical attractiveness, physical agility, physical stamina, sexual expression, creativity, intellectual development, and perhaps self-assurance. This is also the time during which the aging process is taking place at such a slow rate that we may not be aware of any of its consequences.

These few years, ages thirty to forty-five, are the years when our whole body begins to decline. Back in our twenties, the weight of the brain did begin to lessen as nerve cells continued to die. The velocity of transmission of brain messages along the brain's nerve fibers begin to slow down. These changes occur very slowly. Their total effect may be quite noticeable by age sixty or seventy, but may not cause any difficulty in our middle ages. However, many of these changes may not be any cause for alarm.

When we compare the intellectual skills of people age twenty-five and forty-five, we do not find much difference. In some cases, due to their extra depth and breadth of experiences and if their memory is still reasonably good, the forty-fives outshine the twenty-fives.

In addition, aging during the years between forty-five and sixty is still such a slow process that any changes in our brain may pass almost unnoticed by the individual. A reason for this may be due to our expectations about aging during this period. We may just accept the changes since we expect some changes simply because we are getting older. Also, the small adjustments that people make during these years to their own behavior, life styles and self-concept certainly help lessen the overall effects of brain changes. Most often, any sudden or dramatic changes in our brain function are due to serious injury or illness, grief, or major psychological or physiological disturbance.

Studies of mental abilities show a very slight loss in some areas during this forty-five to sixty time period. The vocabulary and knowledge a person has tends to stay constant or even increase. As researchers consider the effects of aging on particular intellectual capacities, they often separate these capacities into two types of intelligence. The two are unspecialized, innate general cognitive ability and specialized, acquired cognitive ability which is based on our many experiences and knowledge gained along the way. Examples of innate unspecialized abilities would be imitating, recognizing oneself, walking upright, sneezing, rules of grammar and syntax, sexual drive, blushing and others that require no learning since we are "wired" for them at our birth. Most often, it is the acquired specialized intellectual ability which remains steady while the innate, unspecialized cognitive ability declines.

Scientists who study our aging population often identify a distinction between fluid intelligence and crystallized intelligence. Fluid intelligence refers to identifying, seeing and using abstract relationships, formations and patterns. It would be used for calculating, architecture, engineering, or playing checkers or chess. This fluid intelligence seems to be less important as we age and in particular for people over sixty since we tend to examine and change our priorities. Crystallized intelligence, on the other hand, has as its source the body of knowledge we have accumulated over time through a lifetime of varied experiences. We use it for assistance in making decisions, choosing from a variety of options, and to form opinions. This form of intelligence keeps on improving and sharpening as we age. Some call it our wisdom.

Other significant information comes from an experiment with age-related changes in persons over fifty. Those subjects were tested on the Thurstone Primary Mental Ability Scale. The longest age-related decline was noticed in logical reasoning found in the left hemisphere. The next longest age-related decline was spatial reasoning found in the right hemisphere. This may be important as recent research has shown that men and women generally use their hemispheres differently and therefore may be affected differently by the aging process. Other parts, such as verbal meaning and articulateness declined less rapidly. These findings allow us to say that even into middle age and later, we are likely to display improved thinking, comprehension, understanding and basic informational capacities.

A variety of sources show that it is very likely that the intellectual and psychological capabilities of persons in later middle age and beyond are strongly affected by the use to which those abilities are put, and the amount of practice an individual gets in using them. Actually, the overall picture of the aging population is very positive. The older person shows all the accumulated advantages of long life experience , wisdom instead of cleverness, and a wealth of accumulated knowledge which seems to compensate somewhat for whatever minor losses there may be due to some neurological and physiological losses or changes.

One of the theories of aging hypothesizes that aging is natural and inevitable and that it is a normal part of our whole life development and process. The physiological changes which begin to occur as we age seem to accelerate as we get older. The senses are less acute, particularly sight and hearing. We talk a little slower as our motor ability lessens. Our handwriting may become shaky and wiggly since the working relationship between hand, eye, and brain loses its precision and efficiency. In addition, during this time period there is a rather noticeable change in our memory as we seem to be less able to remember recent events rather than long-term events. Our "senior moments" begin to occur.

A prominent theory of aging finds its foundation in genetic factors. Support for this idea comes from the fact that long life and acquiring certain diseases show definite family history.

Another important theory of aging is that it is a result of a steady and progressive running down of the body's renewal system. This "running down" may be due to the increasing number of errors that occur in the transcription of genetic information into the proteins which are produced in every cell in our body.

Further strong evidence identified a declining of the normal functioning of our immune system as we age. Through time, our body's antibodies may become changed and therefore are unable to tell the difference between cells belonging to their own organs and those invaders from the outside. These changed antibodies then apparently attack their own body cells as if they were the invaders.

Another major factor affecting some older persons is an emotional one. There is a negative connotation or thought to "old age." Studies have shown that in our Western part of the world that the worst period of worry, despondency, discomfort and uncertainty about the future tends to occur just before retirement. Retirement tends to signal "older" or "old age" and almost "not needed anymore". For many people, retirement turns out not to be as terrible as the individual had feared, especially if the person was looking forward to doing new and different things. Often, at this period of our lives, we must deal with the death of friends and loved ones, as well as thoughts of our own mortality. All together, there are many elements that bring strong challenges to our emotional life.

Since very early in the evolutionary development of

human brains, there has been a very strong and direct relationship and connection of neural fibers between our emotionally charged limbic system, our cerebral hemispheres and the rest of our brain. Research has shown, again and again, that continuous long-term negative thoughts provide much more stress on our functioning cerebral brain than do continuous positive, happy thoughts.

By the year 2010, one out of every six persons in the United States will be sixty-five years old or older and those numbers will continue to increase. According to Richard Restak's 1988 book, *The Mind*, Dr. Peter Davies, of the Department of Pathology at the Albert Einstein College of Medicine in New York City, is convinced that there is a correlation between retained intellectual capacity and the state of the elderly person's brain. Davies says, "I've been struck that some of the brains from normal elderly people over ninety are really indistinguishable from the brains of twenty-five year olds. Absolutely nothing wrong at all. I do not believe there is good evidence for an effect of age alone on the brain."

Evidence seems to point out that for normal individuals a significant number of brain cells die every year and do not recover. There have been some thinkers who believe that this normal brain cell death causes mental deficiencies and senility as a regular, normal consequence of aging. This belief may not be completely correct in all cases.

As we get older there are at least two important factors taking place along with cell death. Most probably, we do lose brain cells every day of our lives. And if we live long enough, we do experience a little shrinkage in the size of our brain. Myelin and dendrites are two factors, which in large part compensate for our brain cell death and allow us a continuing regular brain function.

First of all, the myelin around the axon section of the neuron becomes thicker in a normal healthy brain due to increasing steady usage and good nutrition. The second process is one by which the dendrites develop more branches, thereby improving the communication among all the remaining living cells. The better our brain cells talk to one another, the better we are able to perform the mental and physical activities we choose. We should constantly remind ourselves that there should be, and could be, a steady improvement in some brain functions through the eighth decade of our lives. Changes in our brain functions may not be due to our older age. It may indeed be due to an injury, or disease, or due to our own negligence in not using our brain enough in a positive, helpful fashion.

Our wonderful nervous system changes steadily throughout our life. Since elderly persons make up an increasingly large percentage of patients seen by most physicians, age-related changes are especially important and noticeable. The most consequential of these changes appear in the nervous system. Such changes may start to appear already in the third and fourth decades, but do not usually become noticeable until the fifth or sixth decade with increasing forgetfulness and slowing of some other mental abilities. Perhaps some motor and sensory difficulties show as well. These happenings most often are due to the degeneration of neurons, cell death and the reduction in the number of neurons and in the number of connections at our many synapses. An individual's quality of life is not affected unless the symptoms become serious.

As our brain changes, there are a number of changes which are considered to be universal. The brain gradually loses its size, weight and volume. Over the time between our third and fourth decade to our ninth decade, there seems to be an estimated ten to twenty percent loss of brain weight, depending on the individual. From a number of studies of human brains, it is reported that we lose five percent in weight by age seventy, ten percent by age eighty, and twenty percent by age ninety. The cerebellum seems to lose weight in a ratio proportionate to the loss of weight in the two cerebral cortices.

This brain atrophy is described as a continuing loss of neurons and the replacement of these neurons by fibrous astrocytes, a type of glia cell. Many, but certainly not all, types of brain cells change as they age. Some cells do diminish in size. Their nuclei become smaller and less circular in shape. Some cells that normally contain pigment lose some of their melanin while others pick up a fatty pigment called lipofuscin that they had not contained earlier.

Some of our aging brains will eventually show neurofibrillary tangles and senile plaques. (See Diagram 9) These tangles consist of bundles of tiny tube-like structures that have quickly multiplied and materialized inside a neuron, filled it, and displaced the neuron, causing it to be inoperational. The senile plaques are shapeless forms consisting of granules and filaments which are considered to be a collection of debris or garbage left over from degenerating neurons. This seems to be a chicken and egg controversy over whether or not these tangles and plaques, which are a part of the normal aging process, are due to a disease situation, or reflect molecular misbehavior (free radicals), or could be a part of a serious developing dementia.

A common finding concerning mental change in the elderly seems to be connected to particular changes in some Purkinje cells in the cerebellum. These cells are the main message-transmitting cells in the cerebellum. Careful study has pointed out an estimated twenty-five percent loss of these cells and an apparent similar loss of their connecting dendrites in very old rats. In humans and rats, the cerebellum is highly significant and necessary for controlled movements. The hypothesis is that if this cell and dendrite loss occurs in humans, as it does in rats, it could be the cause of the behavioral and physical movement difficulties we seniors exhibit as we age. For example, controlling a pen while writing, holding a book without dropping it, or playing the piano.

As noted earlier, there are some cognitive processes which tend to slow down as we age. On a test involving speed of response, older people do not score as well as younger people — nor do they score as well as they did when they were younger. The loss of the Purkinje cells and dendrites in the cerebellum may be a contributing factor in this slowing of movement and reaction.

Other than this slowing, it is fairly difficult to list any absolute generalizations about the losses in intellectual functioning for the aged. The variability of "slowing down" among older people seems to be at its greatest when compared to any other part of our life span. Some sixty-year-old people show an observable lessening in mental abilities, while some ninety year olds show virtually no change in their mental abilities, except for being slightly slower in their responses.

There have been some studies that examine the same people again and again over a number of years. The results demonstrate that, generally, the scores on the verbal portions of IQ tests identify little or no decline until the middle of the seventh decade. When compared to the same individual's scores obtained earlier in life, there is almost no change in vocabulary, comprehension, information, identifying similarities, and arithmetic. There is some decline on performance tasks, however.

It may be that age-related changes in hearing or vision cause some part of this decline. For most people, visual and auditory acuity deteriorates as they grow older. The lenses of the eye become stiffer and assume a yellowish coloring. Adaptation to dark may be slower. In addition, there is also a hearing loss and often an increased sensitivity to sounds and speech.

Our aging bodies are also affected by some diseases that may effect our brain function. A major disease is that of atherosclerosis, or hardening of the arteries. This filling up of the arteries affects the blood vessels which provide oxygen and nourishment for the brain. As the brain ceases to receive its vital nourishment, brain infarcts, or injuries, can occur. These injuries can damage and kill brain neurons and its axons and dendrites. Atherosclerosis is a major contributor to dementia in the older population and can cause personality changes as our mental abilities and capacities deteriorate.

The good news is that some research shows that less than five percent of the elderly population — those sixty-five and older — suffer from any dementia at all, while just one to two percent are severely hampered. If and when we are forced to acquaint ourselves with the increasing inadequacies of our brain, we find new ways to deal with our new problems. Our flexible and adaptive brain comes up with alternative solutions — large print books, hearing aids, motorized riding carts, large calendars on refrigerators, special diets, exercise programs, and finding alternate, safer travel routes when driving.

Most often, the brains characterized in the paragraph above refer to normal, healthy aging brains. However, not all of our brains are as fortunate. Plasticity and redundancy, described in the vocabulary section, may not be as functional and significant for everyone as we age. The disease or disorder senile dementia may begin to take over in a fairly slow fashion. The elderly person may begin to lose the memory of events that happened a few months ago, or last month, or just yesterday, or just a few minutes ago. Terms such as disoriented, lack of concentration, clumsy, wandering through rooms and conversations, rambling and incoherent speech, not recognizing friends and relatives, characterize the afflicted person. The standard term for this condition is "senile dementia." Senile dementia is defined by Robert Terry and Robert Katzman as "progressive mental deterioration, loss of memory and cognitive function, with resultant inability to carry out activities of daily living, that occurs in some elderly individuals."

Dr. Mariam Perlmutter, a gerontologist at the University of Michigan, defines cognition in Richard Restak's 1988 book *The Mind*. She includes memory, intelligence, reasoning, decision making and "the representational thinking and problem-solving skills that expand human abilities, enabling us to conceptualize, experience, and communicate with each other." As life expectancy increases, the possibility of a person exhibiting some form of cognitive disturbance or dementia increases as well. In contrast to the good news about dementia shared earlier, other research indicates that ten percent of people ages of sixty-five and over and twenty percent of those over eighty will show significant dementia. We must remember, however, that dementia is neither a natural nor an extreme form of aging. It is a term that combines a collection of symptoms, indicates the presence of the condition, and involves approximately three million people.

Estimations predict that by the year 2010, dementia could affect six to seven million people at a cost of close to $40 billion a year. The worst scenario has many of our elderly caring for many other elderly severely affected by varying degrees of senile dementia. Unless there are some changes made for the care of some of the very elderly persons, they may be in the care of relatives and friends who are almost as needy as they are.

Most recent efforts to study dementia can be attributed to Alois Alzheimer, a psychiatrist at the University of Breslau in Germany, who began to examine elderly patients near the beginning of the twentieth century. He identified the disease that bears his name — Alzheimer's, disease, a degenerative, progressive, irreversible illness that gradually erodes all mental functioning. It may be characterized by faster and faster neuron loss and other particular changes in the brain which results in shrunken cortices and a brain looking neither regular, nor normal.

Some literature says that about fifty-five to sixty percent of all dementia cases are caused by Alzheimer's disease. Of the dementia not from Alzheimer's disease, up to twenty percent may be caused from strokes causing a disruption of blood flowing to the brain and therefore brain cell death. Perhaps five to fifteen percent of people suffering from dementia have a combination of Alzheimer's and vascular disease (difficulties with any of the four main arteries which supply blood to the brain). The remaining ten to twenty percent of dementia cases are due to a variety of causes, such as depression, vitamin deficiencies, thyroid problems, and the effects of one of many medications. Some of these latter difficulties may be treated and reversed.

These days, we have considerable knowledge relative to human anatomy and human brains. There are some aspects which still are clouded in mystery. We are still in the dark about the "agents of aging" and the "agents of human development".

How then is the aging process reflected in the structures and functioning of the brain? And how then are these brain changes shown in our behavior? To date, scientists have more information about the aged brain than they do about the aging one. Many of the changes discussed here have been found in autopsied brains. It is often difficult to identify when certain changes began, how long the changes took, and at what speed they occurred and what was the rate of change. Often, the researchers were not able to determine the long-term health of the person whose brain tissue was being examined.

In one study, brains of people who were judged to be mentally competent when they died were compared with brains of folks who were judged to be suffering from senile dementia. The mentally competent people ranged from fifty-six to ninety-two years of age when they died. While some senile plaques and fibrillary tangles were found in the normal brains, the numbers and total amounts of plaques and tangles were much higher in those people suffering from senile dementia. For the people who were living quite independently and were able to deal adequately with their surroundings at their death, the plaques and tangles were quite minimal in the males and virtually nonexistent in the females. The marked excess of these "abnormal tissue clumps" seems to be closely related to the loss of mental abilities and should not be thought of as part and parcel of a normal aging process or an eventual natural development for everyone.

A neurologists tells the story of an eighty-year-old woman suffering from a minor stroke. She developed a successful plan which allowed her to obtain her release from the hospital. She used the parts of her brain which were not injured to help answer the neurologists questions, "What day is it?" and "What is the date?" She arranged herself so that she could see the clock through a slight shift of her eyes when she was asked the questions.

By getting the information from the face of the clock, she was able to convince the examiners that she was ready to go back home.

Information from a variety of sources shows that the cumulative affects of stress on our brains is not good. Scans of the brains of those who have suffered fairly severe stress over a period of years show a smaller hippocampus than those who have not suffered this kind of stress. The hippocampus is heavily involved in our memory function. Increased amounts of adrenaline are flowing through their brains. The heart and the immune system are affected as the stressful "flight or fight" response causes too much adrenaline for too long a time. The immune system shows a reduction in the number of white blood cells. This would seem to indicate that long term exposure of the brain to "above normal" levels of stress causes reduction in normal and efficient brain function, in some cases through the loss of brain cells due to cell death.

The brain is an exquisitely balanced, dynamically functioning organ. Anything that upsets or alters this lovely balance, especially over periods of months and years affects its normal function and will ultimately seriously restrict its resiliency and ability to recover from damage during its later years.

CHAPTER 8

Five Brain Disorders and Strokes

There are at least five significant diseases or disorders of the brain which seem to occur in our aging population. Signs of these difficulties begin to materialize for some people in their thirties while other people may not demonstrate any noticeable problems until their sixties and seventies. These are Alzheimer's disease, Huntington's disease, Parkinson's disease, Multiple Sclerosis, and Senile Dementia. A brief description of each disease will show its particular relationship to our brain.

Alzheimer's Disease

This disease is viewed by some as an acceleration of the aging process. It is a neuro-degenerative disease leading to brain cell loss. There is some loss of the myelin sheathing around the axons. In addition, there is an excess number of neurofibrillary tangles and senile plaques or amyloid plaques. These amyloid plaques are characterized as translucent waxy substances which are deposited in parts of the brain, clog up these areas, and finally stop the sending of neural messages from one part of the brain to another. Also, lower than normal levels of the neurotransmitter acetylcholine can be observed.

These tangles, plaques, and low levels of acetylcholine are very noticeable in the areas of the brain most heavily related to memory. The abnormal functioning of the affected synapses is probably due to the low levels of acetylcholine, while the tangles may prevent what neurotransmitters are there from reaching the end of the axons. The amyloid plaques seem to block the neural transmission at the affected synapses. These serious disturbances in concert with one another seem to cause a steady degeneration of the affected brain anatomy, in particular the hippocampus, temporal lobe, parietal lobe, and the prefrontal lobe, as the final result is widespread cortical atrophy or shrinkage.

The rate of onset of Alzheimer's increases with age up to about age eighty-five. Age forty is about when the earliest cases begin to show. About seven percent of all people over age sixty-five are said to have Alzheimer's disease. Familial Alzhiemer's disease may be the cause of from ten to thirty-three percent of all cases.

Early effects of this disease begin with gradual loss of short-term memory. Many people perceive this loss as a fairly normal happening attributed to aging. Memory loss leads to an inability to perform typical daily activities — shopping, dressing, eating. Next a lack of self-orientation and trouble learning new information takes place. Some language difficulties may also occur. Personality changes such as hostility and mood swings are not unusual. Some folks then begin to stay away from most social relationships. As the short-term memory difficulties become more severe, all of the problems mentioned earlier become more severe.

The loss of short-term memory severely affects one's ability to learn new information and skills. Solving problems, performing daily living activities, let alone working at a job, becomes nearly impossible. Making good judgments and abstract thinking are increasingly difficult. Speaking, writing, and reading abilities severely decline. Individuals with Alzheimer's are quite disoriented as to their whereabouts and as to day, time, and date. Many patients wander away from home and are lost and confused. Recognition of familiar faces and people seems to vanish as now their long-term memory is greatly diminished. At this stage, most affected people need twenty-four hour, round the clock watchful care.

Severe personality changes occur during these advanced stages of the disease. High levels of hostility, paranoia, anger, agitation, and aggressiveness may be fairly common. Some may strike out in a violent manner. They may show episodes of anger, sorrow, depression, or emotional stillness as if they were not even present.

At the most advanced stages of the disease, the sufferer

may demonstrate nearly no memory nor any intelligence function at all. It seems impossible for the person to talk with others, or do much of anything at all. Awareness of self, others, and one's surroundings seems to have vanished. Muscles either forget how to function or show long-lasting spasms. Bladder and bowel incontinence is very evident. The individual becomes bed-ridden and virtually paralyzed. Death is the final result and seems to occur due to a variety of complications as the body seems to gradually shut down.

The sequence of these serious effects varies a great deal from person to person. The time between the diagnosis and death may vary from two to twenty years. The average length of time between diagnosis and death is seven years. Generally, the earlier the onset of Alzheimer's the shorter the time before death. The disease rarely shows any improvement as it almost always develops at a very steady pace.

Research and analysis of the cerebrospinal fluid, which surrounds the brain and spinal cord, may soon provide the ability for earlier and more valid and reliable diagnoses. At present, only an autopsy of the brain shows for certain that the patient did in fact have Alzheimer's.

A September 27, 1998 article printed in the Syracuse Post-Standard reported that Mark Saltzman, a chemical engineer at Cornell University, has devised a plastic pellet that may be surgically implanted in the brain of

Alzheimer's patients. The pellet, described as smaller than a pea, was placed next to dying nerve cells in rats. The pellet contains a nerve growth factor which encourages the stricken nerve cells back to life. The nerve growth factor (NGF) is released over a period of months. Further exploration of this technique will look at the amount of NGF and the most advantageous time for releasing the chemical into the brain.

Two approved drugs for the treatment of Alzheimer's disease are Tacrine (Cognex) and Donepezil (Aricept). Both of these drugs reduce the levels of cholinesterase, which lowers the amount of the neurotransmitter acetylcholine. Acetylcholine improves neuron-to-neuron communication.

Among the Alzheimer's treatment drugs which are still at the experimental stage are estrogen, Vitamin E, Ginkgo extract, and non-steroidal anti-inflammatory drugs, such as Ibuprofen. Each has its own advantages and disadvantages.

Further in the future are drugs that will also inhibit cholinesterase and boost acetylcholine. Continued study of nerve growth factor will also occur. All of the drugs and chemicals are being examined in hopes that their consequences may be localized or narrowly focused in an effort to reduce unnecessary or dangerous side effects.

Dementia (Senile)

If the loss of intellectual abilities becomes severe enough over a long period of time to interfere with normal functioning, the person is said to suffer from dementia. The most common form of dementia is caused by Alzheimer's disease, in which there seems to be a steadily increasing acceleration of the aging process. Progressive mental deterioration, loss of memory and cognitive function, with resultant inability to carry out activities of daily living that occurs in some elderly individuals are the typical symptoms. Physicians try to be certain that depression is not the cause of the individual's problems.

Dementia is a broad term that seems to describe the situation or state of being that some elderly people find themselves in as a result of the loss of one's intellectual abilities. As the number of aging people increases, so do the number of people being identified as dementia sufferers.

There are, according to the literature, more than sixty different types of dementia. Some types may be lessened and even reversed. These would be dementias caused by drugs, alcohol, malnutrition, infections of the central nervous system, anemia, malfunction or abnormal function of the thyroid or adrenal glands or the liver and kidneys. Forms of dementia which seem not to be reversible are those from Alzheimer's and Parkinson's diseases, those caused by major strokes, heart attacks, repeated head injuries and AIDS. Alzheimer's disease seems to be the source of about sixty-five percent of the cases of dementia.

Huntington's Disease

This disease generally begins in the person's late

thirties and early forties with mild mental problems, especially forgetfulness, along with temperamental behavior, and often with depression. Such behavioral symptoms are sooner or later accompanied by awkward movements, sudden collapses, and uncontrollable flailing movements of the arms and upper body. These movement problems, as well as slurred speech and worsening mental faculties become progressive, leading to total disability and death. The problems described are caused by a degeneration of neurons primarily in the striatum part of the basal ganglia and cerebral cortex.

In some respects, Huntington's disease represents the opposite of Parkinson's disease. With Huntington's disease there seems to be too much of the neurotransmitter dopamine, while with Parkinson's there seems to be too little dopamine. In Parkinson's disease, the major difficulty is the progressive loss of neurotransmitter dopamine in the neurons of the substantia nigra. In Huntington's, the major basal ganglia deficits and abnormal functioning are due to the loss of GABA neurotransmitters in the neurons of the striatum. If we see Parkinson's as a case of functional dopamine deficiency, Huntington's disease may, to some extent at least, be characterized as a dopamine hyperactivity in the striatum. An explanation for these phenomena is that the loss of inhibitory neurotransmitter GABA affecting the message-sending feature of the neurons reacting to the substantia nigra and therefore resulting in the hyperactivity of the dopamine neurons. This explanation seems to be consistent with the notion that anti-dopamine treatments tend to reduce the choreiform, or dance-like, movements. As the disease progresses and the levels of the inhibitory GABA decreases, the inhibition of those parts of our body affected by nerves from the thalamus and brain stem tend to increase the spasmodic involuntary movements which are characteristic of the disease.

Much about the genetic expression of Huntington's disease is known and more and more is being discovered. It is widely believed that the selective destruction of some neurons while ignoring other neurons is related to a neuron-killing process involving excitatory neurotransmitter receptors, especially the NMDA (N-methyl-d-asparte) glutamate receptors. This difficult progress in clinical research is based on the examination and understanding of the physiology, anatomy, and chemical composition of the basal ganglia. This work has been combined with ideas from genetics and molecular biology and gives more hope for sufferers and those predisposed by genetics. In August 1997, the journal "Cell" reported a discovery of what appears to be "the critical event that kills brain cells in people with Huntington's disease." The report states that in 1993, scientists discovered that a mutant gene produces a bad version of a protein. This causes three units of genetic code to get unnecessarily repeated dozens of times. The scientists have now found that this protein, called huntingtin, produced by this mutant gene clumps together in solid cells of "goo" and collects inside the nuclei of brain cells and therefore these neurons are non-functional and eventually dead. The next step, according to plans of the scientists, is to develop drugs which will either dissolve these "gooey" clumps of protein or keep them from forming in the first place.

Although Huntington's chorea is a fairly rare brain disorder, twenty-five thousand Americans are afflicted by it. It is included here because its degenerating neuron feature seems to be somewhat typical of those disorders that parallel the aging process in some people. We hope that a cure or a neuron regenerating factor could provide relief for the sufferers. For now, anti-depressants can help relieve the depression that often accompanies this disease.

Multiple Sclerosis

Multiple Sclerosis (MS) is a widely known disorder in which there is a destruction of healthy myelin around the axons and an eventual near-elimination of that myelin. It is called a demyelinating disorder. The myelin becomes unhealthy, detaches itself from the axon, and therefore exposes that part of the axon it previously covered. The loss of myelin disrupts normal neural transmission which leads to sensory disorders, loss of normal muscle control and slowness of movement. Scar-like plaques settle on the axons where the myelin was once located. The term multiple sclerosis means many scar-like plaques.

An Associated Press article dated January 29, 1998, reported a study discussed by its co-author, Richard Rudicks of the Cleveland Clinic Foundation. The results of the study showed that MS frequently slices right through the axon nerve fibers, in addition to stripping off the myelin from the axons. This loss of myelin and severing of the axon undoubtedly causes our brain to shrink in size. A major problem to be dealt with is that irreversible damage may occur before any symptoms appear to the patient.

Parkinson's Disease

Parkinson's disease tends not to occur before the age of fifty. Its rate of onset seems to increase slowly until age seventy-five, and then its rate of onset shows a slow decrease. The disease strikes men, women, and different races fairly equally. The incidence of Parkinson's has shown to be less than half of the number of either strokes or Alzheimer's disease. The literature describes it as being a leading disease of our older persons' nervous systems. Apparently, it seems not to run in families. To date, the true causes are not completely known. However, due to the changes in the levels of certain neurotransmitters and outward physical behaviors, an accurate diagnosis is quite possible. Although it is considered an older person's disease, it has been known to occur in people in their teens, twenties, thirties and forties.

The disease is accompanied by a loss of nerve cells in a section of the basal ganglia called the substantia nigra.

Along with this loss of nerve cells is a loss of certain brain chemicals, which results in a deficiency of the neurotransmitter dopamine. In other words, the loss of dopamine comes from the death of some of the brain cells as they become dormant or inactive and not functioning properly and therefore not producing dopamine. The basal ganglia, above and near the brain stem, is involved in motor control and movement.

Sufferers of Parkinson's disease display a number of typical and fairly easily identifiable symptoms. Normal function of motor control and movement, attributed to the basal ganglia, is actually allowed through the interaction of several neurotransmitters. Acetylcholine tends to increase the impulses of neural transmission and therefore muscle contractions. Dopamine and GABA act to lessen the impulses and movements. A lessening of dopamine and GABA therefore results in an increase in the regular muscle contractions.

Early Parkinson's begins with changes in the movements of the fingers and hands. One author describes the fingers as seeming to be rolling pills between them. The next development is most often tremors in the arm, hand and leg muscles. The change is in the rhythmic contraction of the muscles that bend and unbend the afflicted joints. These tremors are most noticeable when we are awake, but tend to disappear during sleep.

As the disease progresses, the patient shows muscle stiffness and has difficulty moving quickly and smoothly. Regular daily motions are difficult to perform and take place much more slowly. Daily tasks and necessary job activities become more difficult and eventually impossible.

As normal muscle contractions continue to lessen, facial appearances change. Swallowing and breathing become more difficult. The sufferers move quite slowly and in a stiff manner. They appear emotionless as their faces seem like masks, little emotion is shown, and their voices are very low with little variation in tone, regardless of the topic of conversation. Often, the patient is bent over at the waist and walks with shuffling, slow, painful-looking steps.

There appears to be no cure for the disease nor any way to halt or slow its development. However, there have been some attempts at lessening many of its effects. Among these attempts are giving the patient levodopa (L-dopa), since this drug increases the level of dopamine in the brain. Another effort has been to surgically implant pieces of fetal brain tissue or pieces of adrenal medulla into the brains of Parkinson's patients. These tissues are those involved with producing dopamine. The fetal brain tissue implants have provided remarkable long-term relief to people suffering from severe cases of the disease. The adrenal medulla transplants have not been nearly as successful.

Further recommendations for treatment include psychological support, physical therapy, speech therapy, and medication designed to relieve particular symptoms shown by individual patients.

Parkinson's causes some form of dementia in about fifteen percent of its cases. Some sufferers show depression, mood changes, and loss of interest in their regular activities. Losing one's short-term memory is fairly common. Apparently, these changes are due in part to the disease itself and partly to knowing that one has the disease.

Stroke

Most strokes occur when a blood clot gets stuck in an artery in the brain and chokes off the supply of oxygen to the brain. Damage then occurs to the brain cells. Consequences of the stroke depend upon the amount of damage, the number of brain cells affected, and the location in the brain where the oxygen supply is cut off. Some patients tend to worsen in the days after the stroke. This is due to the breakdown of dying brain cells which releases chemicals that harm surrounding tissue.

Drugs, including citicoline and lubeluzole, are being tested and considered for administration to patients shortly after the onset of the stroke. They seem to attack the free fatty acids and provide building materials the nerve cells need to repair themselves. Citicoline also seems to improve verbal memory of aging individuals. The drug tissue plasminogen activator (tPA) is being used to treat strokes which are caused by blood clots and should be administered within three hours after the onset of the stroke. It helps the flow of blood.

Strokes have a variety of names due to particular causes. There are ischemic, hemorrhagic, hypertensive hemorrhagic, transient ischemic attack, reversible ischemic neurological deficits, and complete strokes. The most common source of strokes seems to be atherosclerosis in arteries of the brain. The arteries seem to become narrow, rough, stiff, and weak due to clogging with fatty substances. The phrase "hardening of the arteries" often fits this condition.

Atherosclerosis may be limited by attending to various risk factors such as smoking, high blood pressure, high blood LDL (low density lipoproteins), diabetes mellitus, inactivity, obesity, stress, type of personality, and high levels of blood iron. Other factors are family history, age, menopause and being male.

The brain difficulties described in this chapter are being studied by researchers from a variety of points of interest. Some of the areas on which scientific investigators are concentrating are genes, chromosomes, the immune system, family histories and tendencies, environmental pollutants, massive vitamin dosages, herbal remedies, drugs which were originally designed for other purposes, and inter-relationships among the items mentioned above. There is more money for research and these results are being shared more readily through the internet and scientific journals. The future for relief from some of the ravages of these problems is brighter than ever before. Our fast growing number of senior citizens may look forward to a longer, healthier "brain life" than their predecessors.

CHAPTER 9

Significant Neurotransmitters

Neurotransmitters are brain chemicals which play an extremely significant role in sending messages from one brain cell to other brain cells. Depending upon the definition used in literature and the purpose of the writer, there are twenty to fifty to seventy or more neurotransmitters. As we age the levels of neurotransmitters crossing various synaptic gaps at the ends of our axons may vary slightly to greatly. The levels of operating neurotransmitters in our brain may influence the way our brain functions and therefore influence our emotional, physical and mental behavior. All is not lost, however, as discussed in Chapter 10, "Keeping Your Brain Healthy" where potential brain difficulties are discussed and suggestions for relief are considered. In this chapter, discussion centers on those neurotransmitters which are of concern to us as we age. These neurotransmitters are acetylcholine, dopamine, serotonin, endorphins, norepinephrine and epinephrine. Also important are histamine, GABA, glutamate, and glycine.

When a signal entering the brain or a signal going from one brain cell to another brain cell arrives at the end of the axon, it causes certain neurotransmitters to be released. These brain chemicals burst forth out of the tiny vesicle sacs at the end of the axon. The neurotransmitters cross the very narrow synaptic gap between their axon and the adjacent inactive neuron's cell body or dendrites, and then lock onto "receptor sites" in that neuron's cell membrane. The receiving cell is then activated and transmits the message to the appropriate part of the brain through a similar message-sending sequence (See diagram 6).

As discussed earlier, there are excitatory neurotransmitters which help send the message on the way to its appropriate destination. Also, there are inhibitory neurotransmitters which restrict or stop the message transmission and keep the messages from moving any further. Some neurotransmitters perform a modulation function which facilitates the excitatory or inhibitory action of such neurotransmitters. At any one particular instant, whether or not a brain cell sends a message, or what kind of message it sends at all, depends on how many signals of each kind it receives and on the neurotransmitters involved in the message sending and receiving process.

To be precise about defining a neurotransmitter and a hormone, and which are excitatory and which are inhibitory is difficult. One author may have the relationship between nutrition and neurotransmitters in mind.

Another author may be examining the behavior of neuro-transmitters in a neural transmission for the purpose of his discussion. A third author may be looking at the human brain and education. A fourth author may be identifying neurotransmitters by their chemical composition and their biological sources. What follows here is general information about neurotransmitters and their task in sending brain messages and how that relates to our aging brains. In some cases, other authors' classification systems are displayed and are used to present a larger picture of neurotransmitters.

By combining three different listings of excitatory and inhibitory neurotransmitters, I have determined for our purposes that the following are excitatory: acetylcholine, asparte (or aspartate), epinephrine, glutamate, norepinephrine, and serotonin. From the same three sources, the following are inhibitory: gamma-aminobutyric acid (GABA), glycine, endorphins, enkephalins, and Substance P. There may be others that fit into these two categories, but we will concern ourselves with only those listed. GABA seems to be the most prevalent inhibitory neurotransmitter in our brains, while glutamate seems to be the primary excitatory neurotransmitter.

As previously mentioned, the chemical diversity provided by all these substances allow our brain cells to exhibit great flexibility and subtlety of responses. One of the most exciting findings in recent brain research has been the discovery that neurons may utilize several neuro-transmitters rather than a single one. This indicates that each brain cell is capable of a greater variety of response than was thought possible only a few years ago. Scientists now believe that this wide repertoire of possible responses provides the basis for our very rich and creative lives.

With the idea of exploring message encoding at various levels of the brain, let us begin with an examination of some of the brain messages. and brain substances that are important for all of us: the proteins, amino acids, and the other modified acids that make up our DNA, our genetic code — the primary message that tells each of us who we actually are.

The main elements of living matter are proteins, which we may compare to the working machinery of an organism. Proteins are large molecules made up of long chains of amino acids joined together. The sequence of amino acids along the chains specifies each protein's physical and biological properties, as well as the actions of the enzymes that govern and regulate life activities. Since proteins determine form and function, they are called information molecules. Their informational content is a function of proteins and depends on the varying number and sequence of twenty different amino acids. Proteins are essential for the growth and repair of our body's tissues.

In a fast-growing embryo, defects or abnormalities in amino acid structure or activity can produce errors or changes in the normal transfer of information that directs the formation of brain structures. Interference with this delicate developmental process can result in severe brain abnormalities. A well-known amino acid deficit involves phenylalanine, which shows itself in the inborn metabolic disorder phenylketonuria (PKU). Two of the brain's most important neurotransmitters, dopamine and norepinephrine, are synthesized within the brain by a series of chemical modifications of phenylalanine. If these modifications are interfered with, a nerve poison, phenylpruvic acid, results. Continued accumulation of this abnormal molecule results in very severe neurological defects and an IQ usually less than 50. In addition, making contributions to abnormal brain structure and function are the reduced levels of dopamine and norepinephrine which result from the absence of the phenylalanine. All in all, phenylketonuria is a good example of an informational difficulty: a disturbance in the coding and decoding of messages.

The next two sections are reprinted with permission from Robert Sylwester's *Celebration of Neurons*. They provide further insight to the function and purpose of neurotransmitters and how they can be affected by each other and various forms of drugs.

NEUROTRANSMITTER SYSTEMS AND RELATED DRUG ACTIONS

Amino Acids

The four amino acid neurotransmitters have the simplest molecular structure of the various neurotransmitters.

These fast-acting neurotransmitters are widely distributed throughout our brain and spinal cord, with concentrations 1,000 times greater than the monoamines.

GLUTAMATE AND ASPARTE: Glutamate (or glutamic acid) and asparte always carry an excitatory message. Glutamate is the principal excitatory neurotransmitter in the cerebral cortex and cerebellum, and it appears to play an important role in vision, learning, and memory.

GABA AND GLYCINE: These always carry an inhibitory message. GABA (gamma-aminobutyric acid) is the principal inhibitory neurotransmitter in the cortex (with as many as one-third of all synapses being GABA synapses), and it's also found in the limbic system. GABA circuits reduce anxiety and relax muscles. Glycine is a major neurotransmitter in the brainstem and spinal cord.

Monoamines

The six monoamine neurotransmitters are chemically modified amino acids that act more slowly than the amino acids. Their circuitry diverges from a single brainstem source or limbic system source and then spreads widely throughout the brain, where the monoamines modulate the actions of the amino acid neurotransmitters. Their actions affect our brain much as a symphony conductor's actions spread to and affect many musicians and listeners. The interaction of a monoamine neurotransmitter with its postsynaptic receptor determines whether the message sent is excitatory or inhibitory.

1. Acetylcholine is distributed throughout our brain, especially in the centers controlling conscious movement — the basal ganglia and the motor cortex. It is the major neurotransmitter at the junction or between the nerves and vesicles and is available at many synapses throughout the brain but most of the neurons that synthesize it are highly concentrated in an area in the lower part of the basal ganglia. As many as ten percent of our brain's synapses use acetylcholine and its action is generally excitatory. It is also involved in learning and memory circuits. This basal ganglia area which projects axons to much of the cerebral cortex degenerates in Alzheimer's disease producing a cortex that contains much less acetylcholine than normal. People with Alzheimer's disease also suffer a depletion of neurons that process acetylcholine in the hippocampus (memory). So therefore, a lower level of acetylcholine certainly contributes to a less-efficient functioning of the brain parts responsible for memory and for voluntary and involuntary movements.

2. Dopamine is synthesized in the substantia nigra in the basal ganglia. It is sent into the limbic system and frontal lobe where its neurons regulate complex emotional behavior and conscious movements. Low levels of dopamine may result in Parkinson's disease and high levels may result in schizophrenia.

3. Histamine operates in brain areas that regulate our

emotions, and its circuitry is similar to that of norepinephrine. It is also involved in allergic conditions.

4. Norepinephrine (or noradrenalin) spreads to a very large number of connections throughout our brain from a very small brainstem structure called the locus coeruleus. It's the primary neurotransmitter for the sympathetic nervous system which has much greater control over arousal, activation, and flight or fight behaviors.

5. Epinephrine (or adrenaline) is chemically and functionally related to norepinephrine.

6. Serotonin spreads throughout our brain from the raphe nucleus cell groups in the brain stem. Serotonin regulates body temperature, sensory perception, and the onset of sleep. Low serotonin levels appear to be a factor in the depression that accompanies seasonal affective disorder (SAD) and various aggressive behaviors.

Peptides

Some 50 peptides (or neuropeptides) have already been identified. They are chains of 2 to 39 amino acids that exert very powerful effects on complex behavior patterns, such as body fluid balance, sexual behavior, and pain or pleasure. Our brain and the peripheral nervous system contain many types of peptides, but each exists in very low concentration. Examples of types of peptides and some actions that have been associated with them follow:

Angiotensin II triggers drinking behaviors.

Cholecystokinin enhances the feeling of satiety after eating.

Endorphin, enktorphin, and dynorphin are a class of opiate-related peptides that reduce intense pain and enhance euphoria.

Oxytocin initiates uterine contractions in childbirth and lactation and enhances bonding between mother and child.

Somatostatin inhibits intestinal secretion and regulates insulin secretion.

Substance P transmits information on bodily pain to our brain.

Vasopressin is involved in water retention, blood pressure, and memory.

EXAMPLES OF HOW AND WHERE PSYCHOACTIVE DRUGS ACT IN NEURAL SYNAPTIC AREAS

1. A drug can increase or decrease the amount of neurotransmitter released into the synapse: (a) Amphetamine and PCP (phencyclidine hydrochloride) increase the release of dopamine, (b) alcohol decreases the release of GABA (gamma-aminobutyric acid).

2. A drug can enhance the binding action of a neurotransmitter to its receptor: valium enhances the binding of GABA to its inhibitory receptors.

3. A drug's shape and electromagnetic properties can be so similar to a neurotransmitter's that the drug can

mimic the neurotransmitter and its actions and effects: (a) opiates, such as heroin and morphine, mimic the endorphins, (b) mescaline and amphetamine mimic norepinephrine, (c) psychedelic drugs, such as LSD (lysergic acid diethylamide), mimic serotonin, (d) muscarine (obtained from a type of mushroom) and nicotine mimic acetylcholine, (e) alcohol and the barbiturates mimic GABA.

4. A drug can attach to a neurotransmitter receptor but not mimic the neurotransmitter's effects: (a) antipsychotic drugs, such as haloperidol, block dopamine receptors, (b) atropine and scopolamine block acetylcholine receptors.

5. A drug can block the neurotransmitter's re-uptake channels: (a) cocaine and amphetamine block dopamine and norepinephrine re-uptake channels (and so extend and intensify the action of the neurotransmitters until enzymes destroy the molecules), (b) tricyclic antidepressants block the re-uptake of norepinephrine and serotonin, (c) prozac blocks serotonin re-uptake channels.

6. A drug can inactivate enzymes that destroy neurotransmitters after their use in a synapse: antidepressants inactivate MAO (monoamine oxidase) enzymes that destroy monoamine neurotransmitters after they have acted on receptors.

7. A drug can modify second-messenger (cyclic AMP) effects and thus change a neuron's firing rate or metabolic activity: (a) Caffeine amplifies and extends the stimulant

activity of cyclic AMP within a neuron, (b) lithium modulates extreme cyclic AMP effects. AMP (adenosine monophosphate) is characterized as another type of neuron chemical messenger. It has its responses mediated or slightly changed by a particular protein. These cyclic AMP messengers can alter the normal expression of our genes and therefore indirectly influence the electrical activity at the synapses.

The above seven items provide a brief look at how drugs may alter the amount and flow of a neuron's neurotransmitters. This, in turn, influences the communication among connecting brain neurons which affect our human behavior with slight to various serious consequences to us.

It seems appropriate to look at another substance that is quite influential in our overall brain function and message-sending. In addition, there has been much publicity in the media devoted to the wonders of this substance — melatonin.

Melatonin has its source and derivation in the pineal gland, a tiny organ in the center of our brain. The pineal gland is the first gland in our body to be formed, clearly distinguishable at about three weeks after conception. The pineal gland synthesizes melatonin by converting tryptophan to serotonin and then to melatonin. Tryptophan is an essential amino acid, one of the building blocks of protein that we cannot synthesize within our body and therefore must get from our diet. Depending upon the definition and sources, melatonin is seen by some as a hormone and by others as a neurotransmitter. Melatonin is therefore the primary messenger of the pineal gland and through melatonin, the pineal performs its many tasks. Melatonin is said to be involved in the aging process, boosting the immune system, fighting cancer, relieving stress, and enhancing sexual vitality. Also, it is described as aiding sleep, influencing jet lag, helpful for seasonal affective disorder (SAD), healthy body nutrition and function, fighting corticosteroids, heart disease and Alzheimer's disease, providing body energy, combating free radicals, influencing our human evolutionary journey, preventing cataracts, protecting our DNA, lessening the effects of PMS, menopause, and helping fertility. Some indications are that future research may look into the relationship of melatonin to autism, epilepsy, SIDS, and diabetes. As with any other interest you may develop in any diet supplement, please consult your own physician before attempting any changes in your daily routine.

CHAPTER 10

Keeping Your Brain Healthy

H EALTHY BODY ... HEALTHY BRAIN; HEALTHY BRAIN ... HEALTHY BODY. Generally speaking, if we maintain a healthy body our brain will tend to be healthy also. There is a very close relationship between healthy, normal brain function and a healthy body, regardless of one's age. Our brain is affected by a great number of factors beginning at the moment of conception. There are factors affecting our brain over which we have very little or no control — who were our parents, injuries, accidents, our early childhood care, and preconception nutrition, for example. Some of the factors over which we do have much influence are diet, exercise, stress, lifestyle, nicotine, drugs, and mental activities. By careful consideration of the factors over which we have some control, we may be able to maintain and even change and improve our brain function throughout our entire life.

According to Mark and Mark in their 1989 book, *Brain Power*, there are four factors which contribute to a healthy brain. The first factor is the physical structure of the brain and its chemical environment. Second is the almost moment-to-moment information received by the brain from the outside world through our senses and from the rest of our body. The third factor is the information stored by the brain from our past experiences. The fourth is the associations or connections developed in the brain between past and present information. All four of the foregoing factors are interrelated and interdependent. In summary, a healthy brain is dependent upon all of these four factors being interactive, and dependent on one another to be healthy and active. A lessening of the activity of one factor may indeed affect the overall health of our brain.

Research studies are taking place about food, neurotransmitters, hormones, nerve tissue growth and repair, mental activities, youth potions, exercise, prayer, vitamin supplements, immune system function, stress, and free radicals. Other scientists are examining loving relationships, dendrite growth, synapses, healing, faith, diseases, surgical techniques, and the aging process itself. All of these studies are yielding increasing knowledge about our aging bodies and brains. The syntheses of all this new information are providing us with perspectives unknown before and therefore providing us opportunities to make changes in our "brain lifestyle."

As we age we slowly begin to realize that aging is no picnic. An older friend once told me that "getting old certainly is not for sissies." However, according to Kathy Keeton in her 1992 book *Longevity* it doesn't have to be a horror show either. She believes that there is really a lot of truth to the old adage that some things, including people, get better with age. The common perception of an elderly person slowly declining into doddering futility is in need of serious revision.

Genes and Human Development

Everything in this section, has been paraphrased or reprinted from *Brain Sex*, 1991, by Moir and Jessel. Our knowledge of human growth and development tells us that from the moment of our human conception, each of us is greatly influenced by the genetic background of our biological parents and all their male and female predecessors or ancestors. We have known some of our human story for some time now. We know that the genes carrying the coded blueprint of our unique characteristics, make us either male or female. In every microscopic cell of our bodies, men and women are different from each other. Every cell of our being has a different set of chromosomes within it, depending on whether we are male of female.

Our identity blueprints come in the form of forty-six chromosomes, half contributed by the mother, half by the father. The first forty-four team up with one another, forming pairs of chromosomes which determine certain bodily features of the "eventual me," such as the color of the eyes, the length and shape of the nose. But the last pair is different.

The mother contributes an X chromosome to the egg (the X describes the rough shape of the chromosome.) If the father's contribution to the fertilization of the egg is another X chromosome, the outcome will normally be the formation of a girl baby. If the father's sperm contain a Y chromosome, normally a baby boy will be born.

However, the genes alone do not guarantee the sex of the child. That depends on the intervention, or the absence, of the other factor in sex determination, the hormones. Whatever the genetic make-up of the embryo, the fetus will only develop as a male if male hormones are present, and it will only develop as a female if male hormones are absent. The proof of this has come from studying people who have inherited abnormalities. It is only by looking at where development goes wrong that scientists have been able to build a picture of what happens during normal development. These studies have shown that male hormones are the crucial factor in determining the sex of a child. If a female fetus, genetically XX, is exposed to male hormones, the baby is born looking like a normal male. If a male fetus, genetically XY is deprived of male hormones, the baby is born looking like a normal female.

In the first weeks in a womb, the tiny fetus is not noticeably a miniature girl or a miniature boy. It has all the basic equipment, such as vestigial ducts, traits, and other appropriate necessities, to develop as either sex. As the weeks go by, the genes begin to put the message across. If things go normally, and everything follows the XY blueprint of a boy, the chromosomes will cue the development of the gonads into testes.

It is now, at around six weeks, that sexual identity is finally determined — when the male fetus develops the special cells which produce the male hormones or androgens, the main one being testosterone. These hormones instruct the body not to bother developing a feminine set of sexual equipment, while at the same time stimulating the development of embryonic male genitalia.

At about the same time, if the baby is female, genetically XX, the reproductive machinery develops along female lines, producing no significant amount of male hormones, and therefore results in a baby girl.

Just as the six-week old fetus was not recognizable male or female in appearance, so the embryonic brain takes some time before it begins to acquire a specific sexual identity. If the embryo is genetically female, nothing very drastic happens to the basic pattern of the brain. In broad terms, the natural template of the brain seems to be female. In normal girls it will develop naturally along female lines. In boys it is different. Just as the male gender depended upon the presence of male hormone, so a radical intervention is needed to change that naturally female brain structure into a male pattern.

This literally mind-altering process is the result of the same process that determined those other physical changes — the intervention of the hormones. Currently there is definite speculation that our human sexual orientation and preference begins to develop as a result of the processes just described.

It has always been a puzzle to the naturally curious why nature should put such a high priority on organizing the sexual machinery of the unborn child. After all, its reproductive mechanism and need is not going to come into its own for years. The answer is that the formation of our sexual equipment is not simply an end in itself. Once formed, the sexual machinery has work to do. It produces those crucially important male hormones. They, in turn, have work to do — on the yet unformed brain.

Embryonic boy babies are exposed to a colossal dose of male hormones at the critical time when their brains are beginning to take shape. The male hormone levels are four times the level experienced throughout infancy and boyhood. A vast surge of male hormone occurs at each end of male development, six weeks after conception, at the moment his brain is beginning to take shape and at adolescence, when his sexuality comes strongly into being.

As with the development of the rest of the body, things can go wrong. A male fetus may have enough male hormones to trigger the development of males sex organs, but these organs may not be able to produce the additional male hormones to push the brain into the male pattern. His brain may "stay" female, so he will be born with a female brain in a male body. In the same way, a female baby may be exposed in the womb to an accidental heavier dose of male hormones and end up with a male brain in her female body.

According to Moir and Jessel, in the 1991 edition of *Brain Sex*, "Ten years ago, most of this thinking was tentative theory. Now it is accepted, to a greater or lesser degree by virtually every brain specialist or neuroscientist." Yet most people are unaware of this fundamental process of life. Hormones are now considered to play a greater role in our early gender development than was thought previously. If most of us do not know that our brains are made differently it is not surprising that we have difficulty in understanding and accepting the differences among people and between men and women.

Implications of Gender

So you, the reader, say "So what does all this brain sex development have to do with aging and keeping our brains and bodies healthy?" This heavy soaking of male hormones, or the lack of it, may be the first early factor which strongly influences the sexual orientation of our brain. This early development could therefore set the stage for the stress and strains the brain will experience the remainder of its life span. Our culture has different expectations for men and women and generally women live longer lives than men. The literature says that men experience more stressful situations and also that women seem to be the healthier and stronger of the two sexes. Throughout their lives men and women, because of their life long tasks and responsibilities and expectations, may need to provide themselves with different forms of nutrition, exercise, hormones, and activities at different stages of their lives.

Research literature seems to show that brain-damaged patients are more likely to be male than female. The supposition is that this situation occurs because men are still taking more risks than women.

Conception and birth rate statistics indicate that about 150 males are conceived as compared to 100 females. However, about 106 baby boys are born for every 100 females.

Generally women are living longer than men, often through their late eighties, nineties, and even into their early one hundreds. This is a reversal of our early history when men lived longer than women.

Men generally have larger brains than women due to a larger body size. Recently it was reported in news articles that men lose brain tissue about three times faster than women from their late teens until about age 45. The cause of this difference in brain tissue loss seems due to the efficiency with which women use their remaining brain tissue. Women are described as being able to reduce the rate of their brain cell activity in proportion to the brain tissue they lose. Men seem to continue using or overusing their remaining neurons at the same or at a greater rate than they did previously. A study reported in the February, 1998 Journal of the American Medical Association reported that women were fifteen percent more likely than men to have tension headaches. As both sexes live longer and longer than even twenty-five years ago, it just seems reasonable and sensible that we should watch over our bodies and brains with increasing care so that we may allow these "extra" years to be as enjoyable and intellectual and challenging as possible.

New and Challenging Activities

A July 1994 Life Magazine article relates information from the UCLA Brain Research Institute. According to Arnold Scheibel, "Anything that's intellectually challenging can probably serve as a kind of stimulus for dendrite growth, which means it adds to the computational reserves in your brain." The major recommendation from the article is to pick something that is diverting, and most important, unfamiliar. A computer programmer could try sculpture and a ballerina might try marine navigation. Brain researchers offer other fascinating suggestions. Do puzzles. People who do jigsaw puzzles show greater spatial ability which is helpful in reading a map. Try a musical instrument. When you decide to play a violin, your brain comes upon a whole new group of muscle control problems to solve. In addition, the brain is asked to function quite differently as the violinist begins to read notes on a page and coordinate the notes with ones fingers to create musical notes and tones. Fix something. It is not only the solution to the problem, but the challenge is highly important for brain function. Try the arts. If you draw well start a diary or make a brief speech to a group of familiar people. Try dancing. Square dancing, ballet or tap dancing are preferred.

Researchers suspect that moderately strenuous exercise helps develop more small blood vessels. Blood carries oxygen, and oxygen provides nourishment for the brain. Again, be certain that the activity is new to you and that it requires thinking. Associate with provocative people. One of the most pleasant and rewarding ways to increase dendrite growth is to meet and interact with intelligent and interesting people. Try tournament bridge, chess, sailboat racing, or group bicycle riding. The article maintains that our whole life should be a learning experience because by continuing this learning process, we are literally challenging our brain and by doing so are building new brain circuitry. This is the way our brain operates regardless of age. It seems almost as if nature intended people to grow more gray matter through new, different, and unfamiliar challenges. Actual new dendrites do appear in our brain as a result of participation in activities which challenge our brain.

Hemisphericity

In Joseph B. Hellige's 1993 book, *Hemispheric Assymetry*, his research among elderly adults, when comparing Performance IQ and Verbal IQ, seems to indicate that the effects of aging may be different for each hemisphere. Some research shows that the right hemisphere may age somewhat more quickly than the left hemisphere. Other research showed a decline in sensory function of right hand (left hemisphere) and a decline in psychomotor problem solving with the left hand (right hemisphere). Still another study showed that elderly adults who relied more on right hemisphere mode of processing information illustrated greater deficits in all aspects of intellectual functioning when compared to young adults and to those elderly adults who relied on a left hemisphere mode of processing information. Also other research has concluded that overall performance on a variety of cognitive and behavioral tasks is more variable in elderly folks than in younger adults.

Nutrition

"You are what you eat." Most people upon hearing or thinking about this phrase begin to consider that it means that the food we eat has a direct effect on the growth and well-being of our muscles, bones, and internal organs. Not many see a strong relationship between what we eat and our brain performance. Well, the latest research points to a very definite relationship between our food and our brain function.

Our brain function relies a great deal upon chemical messengers, the neurotransmitters. In order for the brain to make these chemical messengers from food substances, four things must happen: 1) The substance must be absorbed through the gastrointestinal tract, 2) It must be carried by our blood to a specific area of the brain, 3) It must be converted by enzymes into a specific neurotransmitter, and 4) The neurotransmitter then, must be stored in the proper place, the vesicles, and be ready and available for release when needed. These neurotransmitters have a very powerful effect on our behavior and well being. The various neurotransmitters are produced from different nutrients in our diet. In order for our brain and its neurotransmitters to function properly, it must have these nutrients available to it. The protein we eat is broken down into amino acids. These amino acids, often referred to as the building blocks of neurotransmitters, are carried by the blood to the brain where they are absorbed and utilized in making new transmitters. Lack of certain nutrients can reduce the levels of some neurotransmitters and affect the particular behaviors for which they are responsible. A change in one's diet can positively affect and help solve physical or mental problems caused by particular neurotransmitters. Some of these amino acids needed by our body are produced by our body while others need to come from our diet. Among the sources of proteins and therefore amino acids are meat, fish, poultry, eggs, dairy products, beans, and rice.

Glucose, sodium and potassium play a significant role in brain neural transmission. The vitamins which are thought to be quite important for brain function are Vitamin B6, Vitamin C, and Vitamin B12, along with riboflavin and folacin. Also it is important to note the need for iodine, since lower than normal levels may result in Iodine Deficiency Disorder

Recent attention has been devoted to the nutrition of the elderly, in particular malnutrition. Among the causes of poor nutrition are dental problems, change in our sense of taste, living alone, poor meal preparation, low fixed income, abuse of laxatives, the interaction of food and drugs, and the interaction of the many drugs we may be taking. Programs which assist aging people keep their brains active also help them consider their nutritional needs. The following recommendation for a well balanced body and brain did seem reasonable and reliable: 1) Complex carbohydrates such as bread, cereals, and pasta should comprise 50 percent to 60 percent of our daily calories, 2) Fats should be 20 percent to 30 percent of our daily calories, mainly polyunsaturated and monounsaturated, 3) Eat the freshest fruits and vegetables, as they will retain most of their vitamins, and 4) Eat foods as simple and unprocessed as possible to obtain the maximum nutrients.

Recent research presents information which seems to support that approximately 200 milligrams of Vitamin E enhances the health and function of the immune system in the elderly population. Also noted is a reduced risk of heart disease and a slowing of the steady progress of Alzheimer's disease. One caution described, however, that Vitamin E may upset the effects of blood thinner medication. Interested individuals should consult their own physician before undertaking a change in medication and vitamin consumption. The optimum amount of vitamins, nutrients, and supplements an individual may safely ingest is usually dependent upon age, sex and regular diet, and daily activities.

A February 1997 newspaper report generated by the National Institute of Aging describes the very definite possibility that a decrease in our food consumption may dramatically increase our life expectancy. George Roth, director of monkey studies at the Institute speculates that "people who cut back their food intake (by 20 percent) could add 20 to 30 years to their lives." Roth said it is not yet clear why less food means a longer life. He suspects lower temperature and slower metabolism, due to eating less food, may slow the rate of cell damage that leads to cancer, other diseases, and death. He further speculates that since aging may be due to cell death from free radicals, that since less food is consumed, less food is therefore burned and less energy is created and hence fewer free radicals are created. To date, the Institute's research has involved monkeys, flies, worms, and rodents. These experiments have shown that an increase in the anti-oxidant mechanisms has increased the life span and enhanced the vitality of the subject organisms.

Magazines and television are full of various pictures advertising varied food supplements, such as oat straw tea, barley juice, rosemary, ginseng, cayenne pepper, and echinacea. You should consider these and others in relation to your daily dietary intake as you consult with your physician and a professional nutritionist as the three of you work together for your good brain health. We should not expect peak brain function without giving it the very best nutrition needed.

Free Radicals

Among the ideas which researchers are actively considering relative to the aging brain is the free radical theory. These free radicals are a variety of atoms or molecules that are either lacking an electron or have one electron too many. Apparently they are produced in a strange variety of ways: by heat, air pollution, cured meats, radiation, smoking, dietary fats, asbestos, pesticides, and even by sunlight and heavy exercise.

The imbalance in their electrons makes these atoms highly unstable and "grabby." Since nature resists this kind of instability, free radicals race helter skelter in and around the cells of the body looking for the atoms or molecules which are willing to share. The free radical then combines with its "new friend" and thanks its consenting, electron-sharing partner by damaging or even destroying it. The damage to the cell may range from pieces torn away from the molecule to cutting the cell in half to killing the cell entirely.

By grabbing an electron from the victimized molecule, the free radical leaves the helper molecule unstable and this newly unstable molecule roams around looking for another molecule with which to share or grab an electron and therefore restore its own balance. Now this leaves that next atom or molecule unstable and so on, forming a continuous chain reaction of little disasters which may finally cripple the whole cell. When enough cells have been decommissioned by all this molecular killing, as the theory maintains, the human being begins to get age-related diseases such as atherosclerosis, cancer, Alzheimer's disease and Parkinson's disease. The theory says that the whole body eventually just quits due to all the free radical damage. Theoretically, free radical damage may occur at any place in the body as almost every cell is ripe for attack by these non-discriminating free radicals. Among the aspects of a cell that may suffer damage from free radicals are proteins, fats, RNA, and DNA.

The free radical news is not all bad. Nature seems to be ever alert as we are provided with many substances to combat free radical damage or stop it before it begins.

These substances are known as antioxidants or free radical scavengers. Apparently they combine with the free radicals and turn them into harmless chemicals before they can begin their seeking, sharing, and killing. Some of these antioxidants are said to occur naturally in the human body or perhaps we ingest them. The substances often talked about are superoxide dismutace (SOD), glutathione, macroxyproteinase (MOP), phospholipases, nucleases, glycolases, and calalase.

Strokes and the effects of Alzheimer's disease are among the situations which release free radicals. A study reported in the February 1, 1998, Orlando Sentinel describes a human enzyme which fights free radicals. This enzyme is called manganese superoxide dismutace (MnSOD). According to Mark Mattson, a neurobiologist from the University of Kentucky MnSOD prevents the buildup of the free radicals released by strokes and Alzheimer's disease conditions..

Antioxidants do occur in nature and are available through beta carotene. Sources of beta carotene are carrots, spinach, kale, Swiss chard, pumpkins, apricots, sweet potatoes, peaches, cantaloupe, and papayas. Vitamin E (vegetable oils), vitamin C (citrus fruits and vegetables), and quinines (fruits, vegetables, and probably drinking water) are also sources of antioxidants.

Some concern has been that heavy exercise like running, swimming and bicycle riding and the increased burning of energy can produce bursts of free radicals. A recommendation to counteract the damage the free radicals may do is to consume an antioxidant cocktail consisting of vitamin E, vitamin C, and beta carotene. But only under the guidance of your physician.

An encouraging notion coming out of free radical research is that antioxidants and free radical scavengers may actually slow down the normal process of aging in the brain. Time and further study may provide us a more definite answer.

Jean Carper, in her 1995 book *Stop Aging Now*, claims there are "youth potions" which are ours for the taking. She speaks of our food, vitamins, and our health food store. Further discussion occurs about altering DNA and therefore slowing aging and controlling human destiny and longevity.

Free radicals, antioxidants, mutations, homo-cysteine (a substance in the blood), boosting immune system function, doses of minerals and vitamins, rejuvenating thymus gland function, deficiencies of Vitamin B1 and B12 and use of beta carotene are also discussed.

Vitamin E, Chromium, Zinc, Calcium, Magnesium, Selenium, Garlic, Soybeans, Tea, Fish, Ginkgo, Coenzyme Q-10, and Glutathione are among the anti-aging agents and slowing the aging process possibilities mentioned and encouraged by Carper. She also encourages, as others do, considering these strategies in conjunction with your personal or family health professional.

Immune System and Stress

In the not-too-distant past the immune system was thought to be autonomous, meaning it received no outside control. As a result it was believed there was no communication between the brain and the immune system. Now, there is overwhelming evidence that hormones and neurotransmitters can and do influence the activities of the immune system and that products of the immune system and their interaction are extremely influential for our overall health.

A variety of emotions, thoughts, and feelings ranging from fright, stress, loneliness, depression, control of a situation, anger, love, peacefulness to hate, do indeed affect the release of hormones, neurotransmitters, and endorphins. The brain may literally manipulate the immune system.

One 1996 Stanford University study shows that intense stress may severely impact more heavily on our health than was previously thought. An accumulation of this heavy stress over time can cause brain damage that leads to major depression or eventual memory impairment. People who suffer traumatic events, child abuse, and effects of war-related stress show shrinkage in the hippocampus, a key part of the brain that is related to memory and learning. These people demonstrate high levels of stress hormones called glucocorticoid hydrocortisone. The good news is that lesser aggravations like traffic jams, long lines, being late for appointments, travel, and temporary worries are usually not enough to cause brain shrinkage or damage or may have more subtle impact on the brain than does heavy, intense stress. Some of the studies have shown that, indeed, over time the brain damage that did occur to those in heavy stress situations appeared to become permanent. A working hypothesis for some who are studying the relationship between the brain and the immune system is that stress does indeed release particular hormones and at the same time there is a decreased amount of blood flowing to the brain. This decreased blood flow produces far worse brain damage than what would occur in the absence of these stress hormones. It may be that both the brain and the immune system may be receiving damage from these stress hormones, with the elderly being particularly susceptible in both the brain and the immune system.

As we age, our brains and immune systems, being so closely related and interactive, do show decline in function most certainly related in varying degrees to the length and levels of stress. There are a variety of activities in which we elder citizens may participate in order to lessen the amounts and levels of harmful stress.

Earlier in this chapter, activities that involve challenge and novelty were described. Because of their new-ness these activities could initiate some early frustration and mild stress. As we become more familiar with these new activities, our stress levels should lower as our enjoy-ment increases.

The 1996 Stanford University study pointed out that intense stress does severely affect our bodily health, our brain health, and function of our immune system. Regardless of the source of our stress, there are particular activities that do help lower levels of harmful stress. Among these activities are relaxation techniques, loving relationships, belief in the power of prayer, belief in a supreme being or a God, faith, exercise, faith in healing, volunteering, gardening, cooking, sewing, knitting, read-ing, and crossword puzzles.

Exercise

Exercise can be an excellent way to reduce the effects of stress on our body and brain. The act of moderate to vig-orous exercise releases endorphins, our bodies natural opi-ates, which allows us to have a "pleasant all over feeling." These endorphins are neuropeptides and exert very pow-erful effects on our behavior patterns, in this case, a plea-surable feeling. Rhythmic exercise (bicycling, swimming, walking, running) causes a regular blood flow and oxygen delivery system to our brain. Weight training, which is being encouraged for the elderly helps build stronger and more efficient muscles. The fact of scheduling a regular time slot for your exercise gives you a feeling of being in control of part of your own health program. At the completion of each exercise session there is a sense of accomplishment. Also, a fine extra benefit is that you meet people of a similar interest whom you might not otherwise meet. Problem-solving has been reported by people involved in regular exercise. These people describe how their minds seem to be "free" of their common everyday thoughts and somehow "open to other places" and free of their regular states of being. Then a solution to a problem occurs to them. From time to time, solutions to problems "popped right out" when these individuals did not even know they had problems.

A March 1997 study from the National Long Term Care Survey shows that since 1982 there has been a 14.5 percent decline in the rate of Americans over age sixty-five who are disabled. Kenneth G. Manton says that people are living longer and remaining active because medical science is learning more about treating the elderly. He further states that "They are more likely to preserve lifestyle factors that improve health, such as physical activity and nutrition." Manton also believes the rate of chronic disability will continue to decline for the next 10 to 15 years.

Relaxation Strategies

There are a variety for relaxation strategies available which assist us in reducing the nervous feelings and feelings of anxiety due to stress. Herbert Benson, in his 1996 book, *Timeless Healing*, describes the relaxation response which, in brief, involves repetition of words or phrases and passively disregarding everyday thoughts. Another technique, visual imagery, involves mentally picturing a favorite, warm place while relaxing your whole body while sitting or standing in a comfortable position.

Removing oneself, both physically and mentally, from stressful situations or places is practiced by some. Not going to those places as well as avoiding those situations has been found to be quite helpful. People who practice their religion on a regular basis report it helps them relax and reduce the stress in their lives.

Other activities which help reduce the effects of stress are volunteering, gardening, cooking, sewing, knitting, crocheting, genealogy, watercolor painting, and pencil and charcoal drawing. People involved in those activities report a fulfilling sense of accomplishment and in many cases a strong feeling of satisfaction from doing something for someone else since the products of those activities are often given to someone else.

Ann Sheck, in March 21-23, 1997, *USA Weekend*, lists four "stress-busting strategies." They are Lamaze-type breathing techniques, meditation, new thoughts, and distancing. The two breathing ideas described are "the Darth Vader breath" which involves a mirror focal point for your breath and a cool/warm breathing which identifies cool nostrils and a warm upper lip. The mediation strategy is very similar to Herbert Benson's relaxation response described above. The new thoughts strategy suggests viewing life events in a more favorable, positive light. The distancing asks the participant to put oneself in two places at once by allowing the peaceful self to view the scowling, stressed out self.

Another relaxation strategy which has been found to be helpful is that of massage. It is described by massage therapists as providing relief from pain, muscle soreness and stress, emotional anxieties, and tension. In addition, therapists claim it provides healing energies and body awareness. In particular, massage therapy increases blood circulation throughout the body, and therefore the brain, and perhaps healthier neural transmission. Practitioners believe that our human bodies certainly benefit from the "human touch" in our fast paced, highly technological environment.

Power of Faith

Herbert Benson's recent book, *Timeless Healing* , also discusses the power and biology of belief. Part of the text discusses the notion that faith and belief in a god have been with human beings in all of recorded history, and very probably previous to any recorded history. He presents the notion that our human brains may be wired for God, wired for faith, and wired for belief. Further, he suggests that we exercise this brain wiring by practicing our belief and faith in God, however we perceive God. He discusses various studies which show that both prayer by ill patients and prayer for ill patients seems to have a strong, definite, positive effect on the speed of recovery and the percentage of those who recover from their particular illness. The phenomenon of illness being lessened by prayer has been documented, regardless of the god being prayed to and the ethnicity or nationality of the person praying or the person being prayed for. It is a medical and religious experience worldwide.

Recent Surgical Techniques and Cell Regeneration

Authors Stein, Brailowsky, and Will, in their 1995 book *Brain Repair*, discuss a variety of brain neuro-surgical techniques; the timing of these techniques in combination with other treatments, the site of the injured neurons, brain tissue transplants, brain growth and recovery factors, and the age and gender of the patient. Among the recovery factors mentioned are the environment for the patient, brain function, theories of aging and cell death, the effects of drugs, hormones, and free radicals, physical activity, neurotransmitters, and the redundancy of the brain. They paint a brighter and clearer picture of brain injury recovery, repair, and cell regeneration than ever before.

At another level and less serious type of brain information from Colin Dexter's 1996 novel, *Death Is Now My Neighbor*, two main characters have a brief conversation. While speaking to Sgt. Lewis, Inspector Morse says, "You know something? I reckon orange juice occasionally germinates your brain cells." No scientific or information from Inspector Morse seems to support that notion, to date at least. However, more serious brain researchers have speculated that a lower human body temperature as well as that of transplanted tissue may contribute to the success of some brain surgical techniques.

An article in the March 21, 1998, *Science News* reports a first-time documentation of the creation or growth of new neurons in adult male marmoset monkeys. In addition, the findings support the notion that stress and trauma interfere with the growth of new neurons. Neuroscientist Elizabeth Gould of Princeton University believes that new neurons may be developed by many species, even humans. This new information was initially reported in the March 16, 1998, Proceedings of the National Academy of Sciences.

Laughter and Humor

Since Norman Cousins' books, *Anatomy of An Illness*, 1979, and *Head First*, 1989, numerous researchers have considered humor and laughter as significant factors in the overall well being of the individual. Among the body systems affected by laughter and humor are the immune system, neurotransmitters, emotions, overall brain function, endorphins, pain, and stress relievers. Another feature or benefit of laughter and humor seems to be that of feeling a sense of being in control of one's own therapy and treatment. In addition, there is a strong feeling of being relaxed or a little tired all over that comes after some good belly laughs. Laughter combats negative feelings. Negative feelings and thoughts are not helpful to our immune system function. Our immune system and brain are in close communication. Laughter produces our "good feelings" endorphins. All of these important relationships cannot help but foster better and longer lasting brain functioning.

CHAPTER 11

A Gathering of Thoughts

One dictionary definition of gathering says that the word means "to reach a conclusion often intuitively from hints or through inferences." Another definition says "to bring together the parts of." I would like to gather some thoughts from this book.

In the Introduction I described the genesis of the book, the focus and the audience, and shared some ideas about the nature of the brain and some thoughts about the difficulties inherent in studying the brain.

You then had the opportunity to examine information about the brain through statements about myths, some definitions and aging hypotheses, and important concepts about the brain.

Some details about brain function and neural transmission allowed you to become more informed about the day-to-day, moment-to-moment, and millisecond-to-millisecond operation of our marvelous three pound brain. I hope your appreciation, of what we carry around with us and use all the time, increased substantially.

Information was then shared about some changes which occur as we age. Symptoms and consequences of five brain disorders and strokes were described. Particular neurotransmitters were listed and discussed.

Also available to you were the diagram and the vocabulary sections. In my study of the brain, I found those sources invaluable.

A variety of ideas and strategies for Keeping Your Brain Healthy were proposed and described. As I came upon this information and considered it for inclusion in that chapter, I relied on a collection of criteria. It had to be reasonable and sensible, practical for the user, supported by research and other sources, a good fit to important thinking about our brain, and affirmed by life experiences and common sense.

There are some ideas from Keeping Your Brain Healthy which have become beacons of light or high priority items for me and my current existence. The information about human sexual development was new to me and extremely fascinating. Discovering that new and challenging activities grew new dendrites was quite rewarding and comforting. It seems like an easy thing to do. The nutrition information was quite supportive of a healthy life style. Free radicals and their unbalanced nature and their continued unfriendliness to neighbors seems terrible. It was comforting to realize that they can be obstructed in their task while slowing down the aging process at the same time. The effects of stress upon our immune system and brain was a huge eye opener for me. I therefore found the strategies for relaxation quite helpful. Our family has always been involved in some form of sports and exercise, so that information was quite supportive. I enjoy humor and laughter so those ideas were reassuring too. I am quite pleased that brain researchers and surgeons are attempting to move into uncharted territory as they attempt to repair and regenerate damaged brain cells. They have a significant portion of our future in their hands, eyes, and brains.

Perhaps the notion that was most striking for me is that our brains may be wired for God, wired for faith, and wired for belief. Herbert Benson in his *Timeless Healing* presents very convincing arguments for accepting the ideas that prayer, faith, and belief may be very powerful helpers in the recovery of people from a variety of illnesses. As I have continued to study the brain, I have come to respect the power and versatility of our brain and mind. I am far less quick to dispose of an idea that initially seems to be foolish, strange, and unreasonable. I find it quite fascinating to consider the possibilities of prayer.

So what does this all mean? A February 15, 1998 newspaper article discusses "Aging redefined." The article describes Americans in the seventies and eighties as being at the vanguard of "The Third Age" or "the extension of healthy middle age" well into our seventies, eighties, and nineties. This third age is attributed to much better health habits, near elimination of near fatal diseases (polio, tuberculosis, scarlet fever), and a discovery of a way to reverse cellular aging.

It seems to me that if individuals pay attention to what is available to them through news articles, television, books, seminars, community news letters, magazines, and course work they could develop a healthy brain lifestyle. This style of living and caring and studying and attending could give them twenty to forty more years of active life than was anticipated. Lydia Bronte, director of The Aging Society Project for the Carnegie Corporation, sees these years as "part of a normal adulthood rather than of old age." If we intend to enjoy these years, it seems imperative that we try to develop and maintain a healthy brain. I believe we have the information to do just that. On May 27, 1998 News Service Reports proclaimed that people in nearly all countries of the world are living decades longer than generations born in the previous century. A conference held in Paris, France and organized by the International Council for Global Health Progress described the subsequent changes due to this increased life span have been rapid, dramatic, and revolutionary. Researchers pointed out that by the year 2050, nearly one fifth of the world's populations will be over the age of 65 compared with one percent in the year 1900. There will be large numbers of people living decades after the current retirement ages. Adaptations will have to be made in economics, family roles, medicine, housing, and lifestyle. If *Our Aging Brain: Changing and Growing* has allowed you to look at your own personal brain-style, then I believe a contribution has been made.

Appendix I

DIAGRAMS

1. Top view of two hemispheres.

2. Three dimensional view from left rear.

3. Side view of left and right hemispheres.

4. Right Hemisphere, inside center.

5. Neural circuit.

6. Synapse area (axon, synapse, dendrite).

7. View of normal neurons in the cerebellum.

8. View of neurons in aging brain.

9. Senile plaques and fibrillary tangles-
   Alzheimer's' patient.

DIAGRAM 1

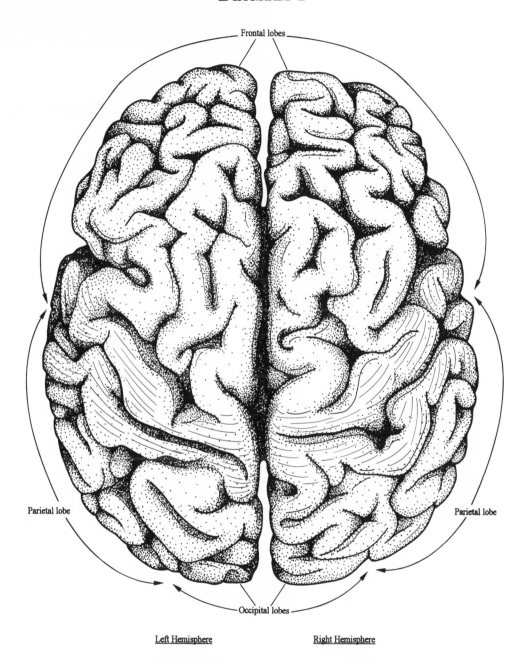

Frontal lobes

Parietal lobe

Parietal lobe

Occipital lobes

<u>Left Hemisphere</u>

<u>Right Hemisphere</u>

This is a top view of the brain (three-quarters actual size). The two hemispheres and three lobes are identified. The temporal lobe is identified on Diagram 3.

Source: *Brain, Mind and Behavior*, 1988 by Bloom and Lazerson
W. H. Freeman and Company

DIAGRAM 2

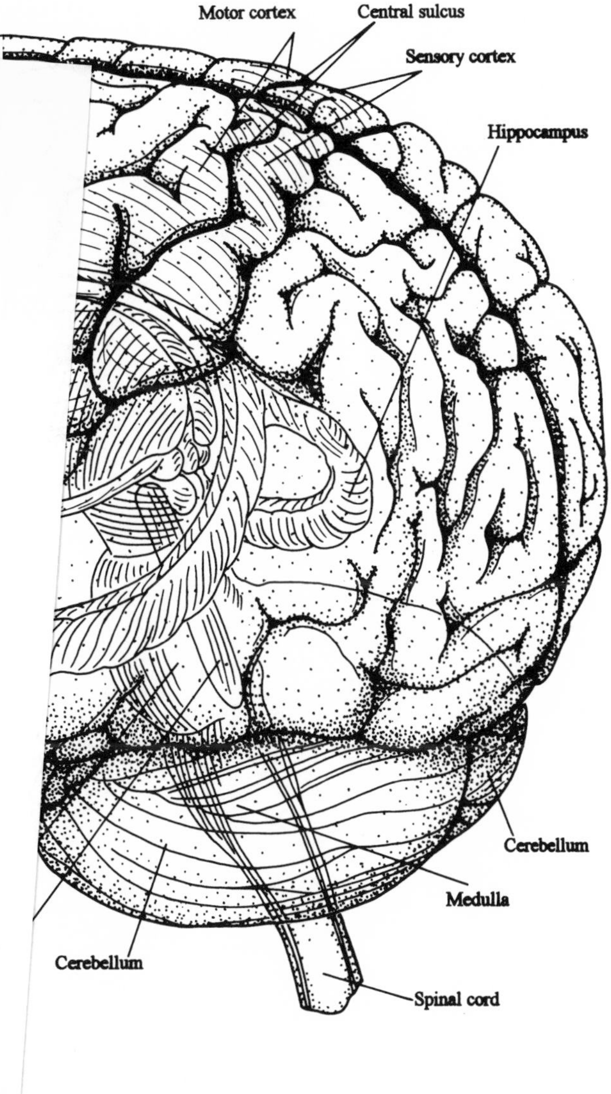

Motor cortex

Central sulcus

Sensory cortex

Hippocampus

Cerebellum

Medulla

Cerebellum

Spinal cord

...nal view of the brain seen from the left

...nd and Behavior, 1988 by Bloom and Lazerson
W. H. Freeman and Company

DIAGRAM 3

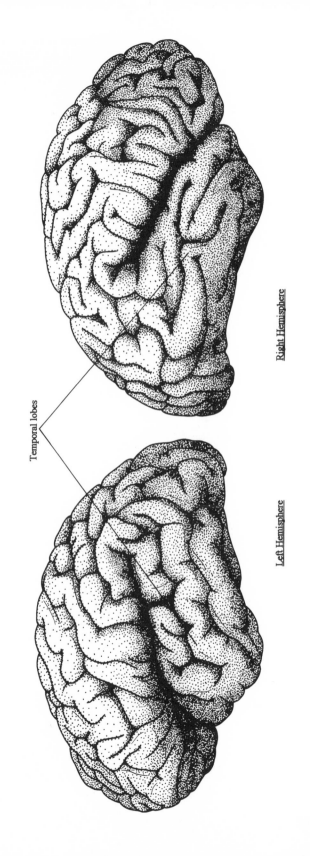

Temporal lobes

Left Hemisphere

Right Hemisphere

This diagram shows an outside view of the left and right hemispheres.

Source: *Brain, Mind and Behavior*, 1988 by Bloom and Lazerson
W. H. Freeman and Company

Diagram 4

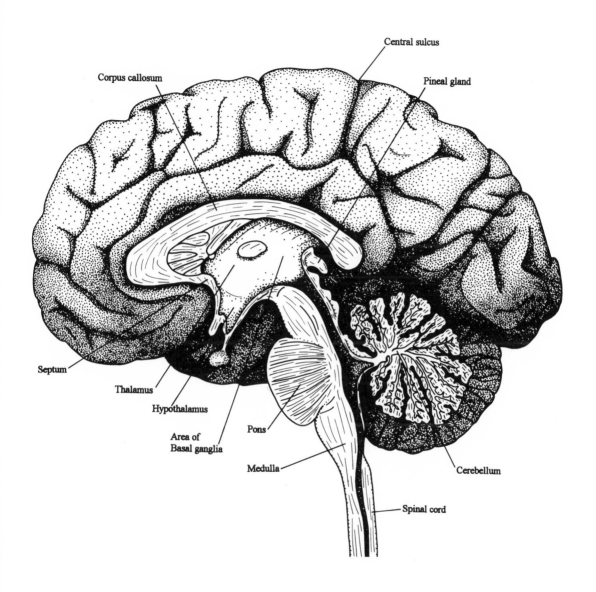

Shown here is a view of the right hemisphere as it would appear if the brain was cut right down through the midline between the two hemispheres.

Source: *Brain, Mind and Behavior*, 1988 by Bloom and Lazerson
W. H. Freeman and Company

DIAGRAM 5

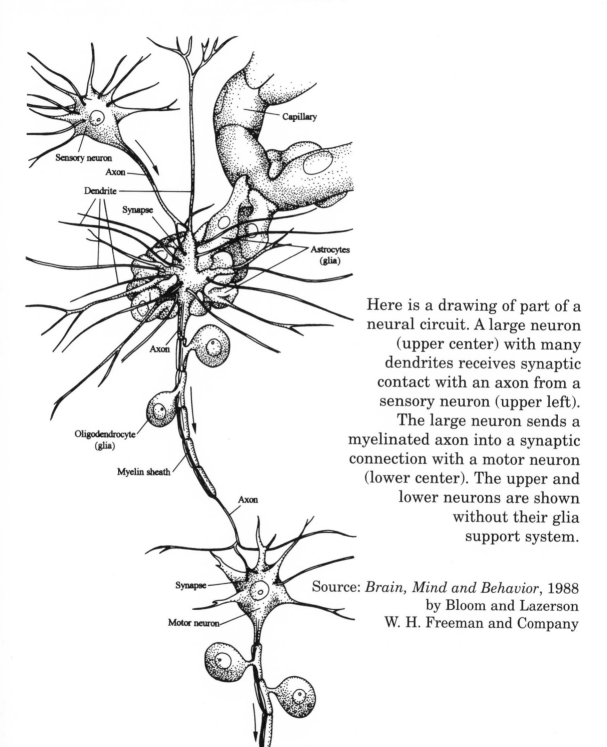

Capillary

Sensory neuron

Axon

Dendrite

Synapse

Astrocytes
(glia)

Axon

Oligodendrocyte
(glia)

Myelin sheath

Axon

Synapse

Motor neuron

Here is a drawing of part of a neural circuit. A large neuron (upper center) with many dendrites receives synaptic contact with an axon from a sensory neuron (upper left). The large neuron sends a myelinated axon into a synaptic connection with a motor neuron (lower center). The upper and lower neurons are shown without their glia support system.

Source: *Brain, Mind and Behavior*, 1988
by Bloom and Lazerson
W. H. Freeman and Company

DIAGRAM 6

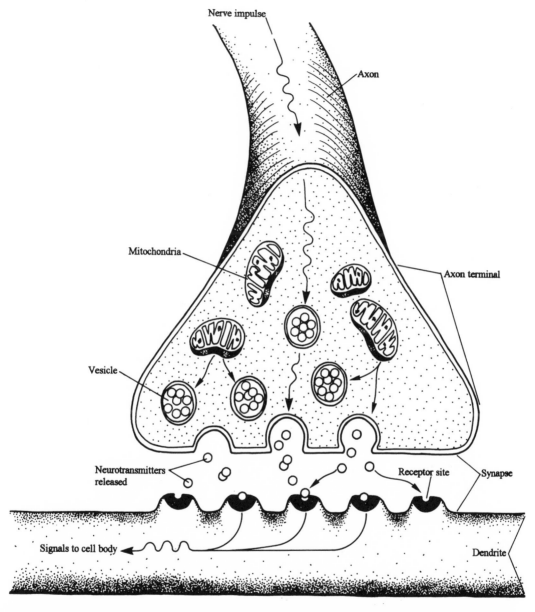

Nerve impulse

Axon

Mitochondria

Axon terminal

Vesicle

Neurotransmitters released

Receptor site

Synapse

Signals to cell body

Dendrite

Shown here is an enlarged view of a synaptic area where an axon almost touches a dendrite.

Source: *A Celebration of Neurons,* 1995 by Robert Sylwester, A.S.C.D.

DIAGRAM 7

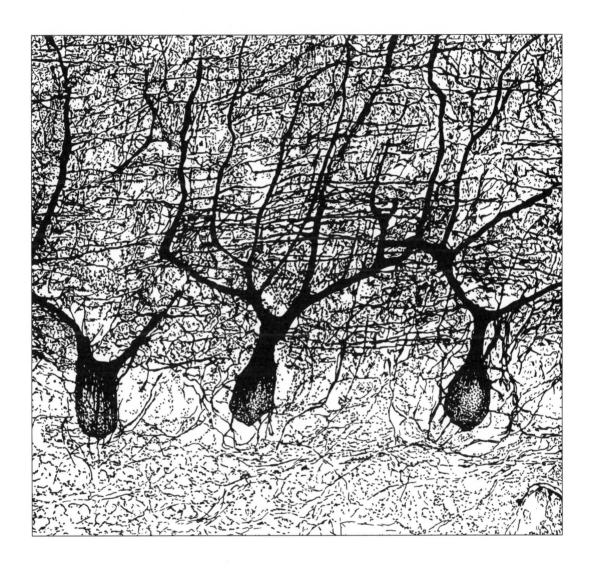

This diagram shows healthy neurons in the cerebellum. Pictured are the cell body, axon and numerous dendrites.

Source: *The Mind*, 1988 by Richard M. Restak,
Educational Broadcasting Corporation

DIAGRAM 8

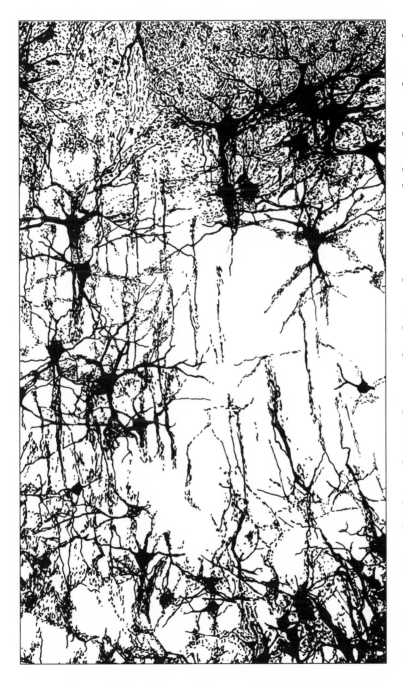

As a person ages the branching of many dendrites decreases and therefore reduces the connections and communication between neurons. The "empty spaces" indicate the loss of dendrites.

Source: *The Mind*, 1988 by Richard M. Restak
Educational Broadcasting Corporation

DIAGRAM 9

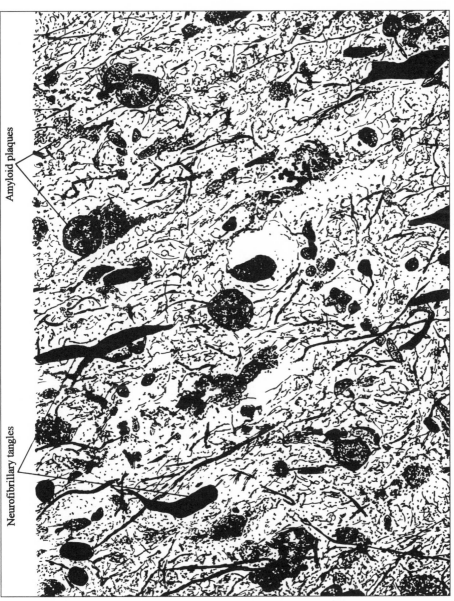

This illustration shows senile plaques, or masses of beta-amyloid protein, and fibrillary tangles in the brain of an Alzheimer's victim. Normal degenerating neurons often appear darker than healthy neurons.

Source: *The Mind*, 1988 by Richard M. Restak
Educational Broadcasting Corporation

Appendix II

<u>Vocabulary</u>

The following information is organized into two sections. The first section is provided for those who would like a very basic understanding of brain anatomic terminology, and therefore, could read the text fairly easily. The terms listed in this section are labeled on at least one of the diagrams numbered one through six.

The second section is for those who would like a more thorough understanding of brain anatomy and function. I found the vocabulary included in the two sections significant and important in my study of the brain. As you will notice, some of the items are explained more extensively than others because I found those definitions quite interesting, informative, and helpful in bringing many ideas together.

Section 1

neuron: the individual nerve cell, the building block of the brain. Each neuron sends nerve impulses over a single long fiber (the axon) and receives nerve impulses over numerous short fibers (the dendrites). There are billions of neurons in the human brain. Some literature says that there is the potential for one trillion neurons to exist.

axon: a single axon extends away from the neuron and provides the pathway over which signals can travel from the cell body for long distances to other parts of the brain and nervous system and to muscles and glands. Axons join dendrites and cell bodies of other neurons at synapses.

dendrite: the purpose of the dendrites of a neuron is to increase the surface of a neuron and therefore increase the influence of neurons on each other. Dendrites bring information to the neuron.

myelin: exists as many dense layers of "insulation" wrapped around each axon during the development of the embryo. The myelin exists in sections. The myelin sheath helps signals and nerve impulses travel along the axon. Nerve impulses travel faster over myelinated axons than they do over unmyelinated fibers or nerve fibers with poorly developed myelin. Myelin develops normally in a healthy brain as both hemispheres are used in an active and a complementary manner.

glia cells: "nerve glue," special cells that surround each neuron, providing support and nourishment. There are many more glial cells than there are neurons.

synapse: a unique bumpy, button-like structure and tiny space which connects axons to dendrites, also from axon to axon and axon to cell body. A typical neuron may have 1,000 to 10,000 synapses and may receive signals or impulses from 1000 other neurons. Each synapse can be considered a component of an inside world where neurons interact with each other in ways dependent on the brain's developmental history, its experiences, the richness of the outside environment, and the variety and complexity of sensory experiences. Throughout life — not just during the first few months — the brain's synaptic organization can be changed by its various interactions with its environment, both inside and outside.

neurotransmitters: chemicals liberated by neurons which cause electrical charges to be transmitted across the synapse (gap) between nerve cells. Neurotransmitters thus control the message given to, and received by, all the cells and systems of the body.

corpus callosum: the main connecting tissue between the two brain hemispheres which consists of 200 million or more nerve fibers. The nerve fibers carry information both ways allowing the two hemispheres to "talk to each other". It may not be completely developed until around age ten.

frontal lobe: the frontal lobe lies directly behind the forehead. The hind-most part of this lobe contains the motor cortex but the function of the remaining portion is somewhat unclear. Some researchers theorize that foresight, planning, and personality are located in the prefrontal lobe.

temporal lobe: the area of the cerebral cortex located near the temples of the skull that contains centers for hearing and memory and language.

parietal lobe: contains sensory cells that respond to heat, touch, cold, pain, and body position which cluster in parallel ribbons of nerve tissue behind the central sulcus. Association areas in the parietal lobe are thought to synthesize information from the somatosensory cortex — messages from the skin, muscles, tendons, and joints about the body's position and movement along with information about sight and sound transmitted from the visual and auditory cortices in the occipital and temporal lobes.

occipital lobe: the visual cortex occupies an area in the occipital lobe, at the back of each hemisphere. From the retinas, light triggered impulses race over the million fibers of the optic nerve, half of them crossing at the chiasm junction in front of the brainstem. They fan out through twin clusters called lateral geniculate bodies, and, traveling at speeds of up to 400 feet per second, rush into the occipital cell bank, stimulating the miracle of seeing.

SECTION 2

amygdala: deep in the forebrain lies the amygdala, a walnut-sized mass of gray cells. Animal experiments have shown that it is active in the production of aggressive behavior or fear reactions. Each one is a mass of nerve cells thought to be related to feelings of rage and aggression. Every memory stimulus has a more or less indirect pathway by which it connects with two areas of the brain we believe are most important in memory, the amygdala and hippocampus.

atrophy: the wasting away or shrinking of tissues or organs often due to lack of usage or in some cases through the natural aging process.

basal ganglia: a collection of nerve cells (ganglia) at the base of the cerebral cortex in each hemisphere above the pons and lateral to the thalamus. (Included in this collection are the caudate nucleus, putamen, globus pallidus, subthalamic nucleus, and substantia nigra.) These nerve cells, in conjunction with the thalamus, cerebral cortex, and cerebellum, regulate specific, complex, reflexive motor movements, such as starting, slowing, stopping. The basal ganglia have been identified as having some relationship to Tourette's Syndrome, Obsessive-Compulsive Disorder, Parkinson's Disease, the Savant Syndrome, and Huntington's Disease.

canalization: to channel into a particular direction, the tendency of any organic system like the nervous system seems to follow certain developmental paths rather than others. "Indeed, the nervous system grows in an exquisitely timed and elegantly programmed fashion." (see also plasticity and redundancy).

cerebellum: a relatively large structure attached to the back of the brain. Its intricate cellular architecture helps control movement by connections to the pons, medulla, spinal cord, and thalamus.

cerebral cortex: the largest part of the brain. It is the outer layer of the brain, about one-eighth of an inch thick, which covers the two hemispheres consisting of the frontal, temporal, parietal, and occipital lobes.

downshifting: when the individual detects threat or fear or embarrassment in an immediate situation, full use of the great, new cerebral brain is suspended, and faster acting, simpler older brain resources take larger roles. (see Triune Brain)

fornix: the two-way communicating fiber system of axons connecting the hypothalamus and the hippocampus.

hippocampus: U-shaped formations in the limbic system, thought to play an important role in learning and converting short-term memory to long term memory. These hippocampal formations are often affected negatively by Alzheimer's Disease.

homeostasis: a state of psychological and physiological equilibrium produced by a balance of functions and of chemical composition within an organism.

hypothalamus: nestled between the thalamus above and the brainstem below, lies a small cluster of nerve cells called the hypothalamus. Only the size of a thumb tip, its blood supply is one of the richest in the entire body. From it arise feelings of pleasure, punishment, hunger, thirst, sexual arousal, aggression, and rage.

Through its connection with the brainstem, the hypothalamus maintains homeostasis, the body's internal equilibrium. It keeps body temperature at roughly 98.6 degrees by means of a complex thermostat system that reacts to messages from temperature- sensing skin receptors and impulses from heat-sensitive nerve cells near the front of the hypothalamus.

Hunger and thirst centers in the hypothalamus serve as the body's appestate. Here, tiny receptors, sense organs, trace glucose levels in the blood. When supplies of this vital energy food plummet, the hypothalamus generates hunger pangs. Hypothalamic disorders may cause compulsive eating or loss of interest in food, depending on the particular hypothalamic region affected. The sensation of thirst arises through receptors measuring the salt levels in the blood. With this sophisticated sensing system, the body balances and replenishes itself.

lateral geniculate nucleus: two sets of nerve cells or neurons which receive visual information through and from the optic tract and carry it back to the visual cortex. They are located near the superior colliculus and thalamus.

lateralization: the tendency to use one hemisphere more than the other. Persons who are lateralized move almost totally to using the right hemisphere or to using the left hemisphere, depending on the task.

medulla oblongata: the brain region between the pons and the spinal cord that operates as a control center for respiration, blood pressure, and heart rhythm.

mixed dominant: someone who has refined talents in both hemispheres and the ability to shift appropriately, depending on the task, between the two hemispheres.

nucleus: 1) collections of nerve cell bodies; 2) often called the information center of the cell. The nucleus of each cell holds all the genes that make up the chromosomes.

nucleus accumbens: a small area in the center of the frontal lobe which receives information from the neocortex, the basal ganglia, and the limbic system (in particular, the hippocampus and the amygdala).

optic chiasm: area where the optic nerves from each eye come together and some fibers cross over to the opposite hemisphere of the brain. It is located at the base of the front of the hypothalamus.

pathologic: pertaining to a difficulty of behavior caused by a disease.

pineal gland: Seventeenth century Rene Descartes singled out the pineal gland, a tear drop of flesh in the back of the brain, as "the seat of consciousness." It is located below the back end of the corpus callosum.

One of the products of this tiny gland, located deep in the center of the brain, is the hormone melatonin. Acting on information received from the eyes about the photo period — the light-dark cycle — the pineal gland secretes melatonin during the hours of darkness. This hormone is now known to be heavily involved in both seasonal and daily rhythms. Research is underway to see how melatonin can be used to combat conditions such as depression, jet lag, and sleep disorders, as well as a number of other significant areas of human interest. In a number of non-human animals, the pineal gland seems to serve as a light influenced biological clock.

pituitary gland: is situated below its controlling organ, the hypothalamus. This gland secretes hormones which regulate other endocrine glands, controlling growth, reproduction, and numerous metabolic processes. Some have called it the body's "master gland."

When sensors in the hypothalamus detect a drop in hormones in the blood stream, the hypothalamus instructs the pituitary to step up production. It is a delicate system of reciprocity. Through sexual arousal, hormones act directly on the hypothalamus which, in turn, orders the actions of the pituitary. So crucial is it in regulating sexual impulses that injury to certain hypothalamic regions can kill the sex urge entirely.

plaques: degenerated networks of nerve cell terminals found in the brains of those who have died of Alzheimer's Disease. These plaques (senile) seem to go hand-in-hand with black fibrillary tangles which fill many of the neurons of Alzheimer's patients.

plasticity: a reference to the considerable flexibility in human growth and development of the brain, especially during the early months of life. (see also canalization and redundancy)

pons: a part of the brain stem that works in conjunction with the medulla, hypothalamus, and thalamus to control respiration and heart rhythms. The pons is the major route by which the forebrain sends information to and receives information from the spinal cord and peripheral nervous system.

protein: see Significant Neurotransmitters chapter.

redundancy: we are born with far more brain neurons than we will ever need or ever use. This feature of our human development is extremely helpful as we may lose about 18,000,000 brain cells each year.

reticular activating formation: a zone of extended structures within the pons and medulla that play an important role in arousal (sleep and wakefulness) and attention. Its nonspecific neurons (not sensory, not motor) receive sensory information from various neural sources and act as a filter, passing on only information that is novel and persistent.

senescence: growing old, aging, exhibiting signs of senility, worn away nearly to the basic level, at the end of a cycle.

septum: a thin, triangular membrane in the brain connected to the hypothalamus; believed to contain nerve centers for pleasure.

superior colliculi: collection of nuclei located near the top of the brain. They function as a relay station in the visual system, along with the integration of information used in spatial organization and perception of motion. They are tucked in below the thalamus.

thalamus: almost all information must pass through the thalamus on the way to and from the overarching cerebral hemispheres. Each of the senses, except smell, relays its impulses through the thalamus. They are a twin-lobed mass of nerve cells at the top of the brainstem containing relay centers for sensory and motor information to and from the brain. The two thalami, side-by-side domes, at the top of the brainstem help to regulate consciousness. Gray masses packed in the domes gather information from nearly every area of the body, relaying sensory impulses to the cerebrum above.

triune brain: Paul D. MacLean's explanation represents his view of the evolutionary development of our brain structure over the last 250 million or so years. His explanation calls the oldest brain the "reptilian brain." The second brain to evolve is called the old "mammalian brain," while the third and youngest brain is labeled the "neomammalian brain." Each of the brains serves general and particular purposes and functions. Each of the three brains is chemically different from the other two, but do communicate with the other two.

ventricle: small anatomical cavities or spaces of the brain filled with clear, colorless cerebrospinal fluid as it circulates through and around the brain and spinal cord.

vesicle: little packets of different sizes and shapes at the end of an axon terminal, where neurotransmitters are stored as they wait to be released into the synapse during neural transmission of brain information.

Appendix III

<u>TWENTY FIVE MYTHS OR MISCONCEPTIONS</u>

F 1) There is no scientific support for the relationship between the size of one's head and the size of the brain.

T 2) There is some published support for the idea that eating fish and fish oil will improve our brain function by regulating neurotransmitters and stress hormones.

T 3) The popular and scientific literature reports that we do indeed use only about ten percent of our brain capacity.

F 4) We tend to use both our hemispheres for much of what we ask our brain to do for us. Some people, due to serious epilepsy difficulty, do have one of their hemispheres surgically removed. See item number 16.

F 5) As we age our brain does change and we may notice difficulties we have not experienced before. However, particular brain functions do not diminish and may even improve.

F 6) Smoking, alcohol, and certain drugs kill brain cells which might otherwise continue to live and function.

F 7) Both of the brain diseases, Alzheimer's and Multiple Sclerosis, may affect people in their late thirties and early forties.

F 8) The incidence of strokes may be reduced by a healthy lifestyle involving at least nutrition, exercise and stress reduction.

F 9) The brains of men begin to age at an earlier age than women, but women tend to catch up later on.

F 10) The food we eat has a great effect on the overall health of our brain. There are certain foods we must have for normal brain function.

F 11) Depending on the particular type of "forgetfulness" we are experiencing, there are a number of adjustments we can make to counteract that phenomenon.

T 12) Please see the Triune Brain in the vocabulary sections of Appendix II.

T 13) Men, due to larger body size, have brains which are about ten percent larger. Women are described as using their brains more efficiently.

T 14) Scientists have verified that our brain cells begin to die moments after we are born.

T 15) Yes, longevity studies support a twenty percent loss in weight and size.

T 16) The operation is called a hemispherotomy or a hemsipherectomy.

T 17) Scientists, aided by modern technology, support this blood flow amount.

T 18) Sadly, that is the situation today.

T 19) That is a true statement, even though our brain takes up far less than twenty percent of the body's space.

T 20) Those who study our human evolutionary development seem to agree on that point. See the response to Item Number 12.

T 21) Physicians seem to agree that it is the ravages inflicted on the brain and body by the disease that ultimately kills the patient.

F 22) Research reports that the earlier the onset of Alzheimer's disease, the speedier the death of the patient.

T 23) Some philosophers maintain that our brains were appropriate for a far simpler culture and have not evolved fast enough to keep up with the changes in our human culture. We continue to struggle with such problems as air and water pollution, destruction of rain forests, cloning, human relationships, and the homeless.

F 24) There is no scientific support of this statement.

F 25) Most authors and researchers maintain that our brain development is a function of both genetic make up and our environment.

Appendix IV

If You Need More Information

If after reading *Our Aging Brain: Changing and Growing*, you need more clarification about something or you wish for more information about a particular topic, perhaps I may be able to help you.

Should you wish to contact me, please send your written questions to me at the address listed below. Include your phone number and a self-addressed stamped envelope. I do have a number of sources available to me, human, text and the Internet.

Harold W. Nash
P.O. Box 3293
Burlington, NC 27215-0293

Bibliography

Albom, M. (1997). *Tuesdays with Morrie*. New York, N.Y., Doubleday.

American College Dictionary (1985). Boston, Mass., Houghton Mifflin.

Armstrong, T. (1987). *In Their Own Way*. Los Angeles, Calif., Tarcher.

Benson, H. (1996). *Timeless Healing*. New York, N.Y., Scribner.

Bloom, F. and Lazerson, A. (1988). *Brain, Mind, and Behavior*. New York, N.Y., Freeman.

Blum, D. (1997). *Sex On The Mind*. New York, N.Y., Viking Penguin.

Calvin, W. (1996). *How Brains Think*. New York, N.Y., Basic Books.

Canter, M. (1996). *Ember From The Sun*. New York, N.Y., DelaCorte Press.

Carper, J. (1995). *Stop Aging Now*. New York, N.Y., HarperCollins.

Carter, J. (1998). *The Virtues of Aging*. New York, N.Y., Ballantine.

Cooper, J., Bloom, F. and Roth, R. (1996) *The Biochemical Basis of Neuropharmacology*. New York, N.Y., Oxford University Press.

Cousins, N. (1989). *Head First, The Biology of Hope*. New York, N.Y., Dutton.

Cousins, N. (1979). *Anatomy Of An Illness*. New York, N.Y., Bantam Press.

De Armond, S., Fusco, M. and Dewey, M. (1989). *Structure of the Human Brain*. New York, N.Y., Oxford University Press.

Diamond, J. (1992). *The Third Chimpanzee*. New York, N.Y., HarperCollins.

DiGiovanna, A. (1994). *Human Aging: Biological Perspectives*. New York, N.Y., McGraw-Hill.

Gardner, H. (1985). *Frames of Mind*. New York, N.Y., Basic Books.

Gazzaniga, M. (1992). *Nature's Mind*. New York, N.Y., Basic Books.

Harth, E. (1990). *Dawn of a Millenium*. Boston, Mass., Little, Brown & Co.

Haas, R. (1994). *Eat Smart, Think Smart*. New York, N.Y., HarperCollins.

Hayflick, L. (1994). *How and Why We Age*. New York, N.Y., Ballantine Books.

Heimer, L. (1995). *Human Brain and Spinal Cord*. New York, N.Y., Springer-Verlag.

Hellige, J. (1993). *Hemispheric Assymetry*. Cambridge, Mass. Harvard University Press.

Hobson, J. (1988). *The Dreaming Brain*. New York, N.Y., Basic Books.

Keeton, K. (1992) *Longevity*. New York, N.Y., Viking Press.

Langston, J. and Palfreman, J. (1995). *The Case of the Frozen Addicts*. New York, N.Y., Parthean.

Maguire, J. (1990). *Care and Feeding of the Brain*. New York, N.Y., Doubleday.

Mahoney, D. and Restak, R. (1998). *The Longevity Strategy*. New York, N.Y., Wiley.

Mark, V. and Mark, J. (1989). *Brain Power*. Boston, Mass., Houghton Mifflin.

Medina, J. (1996). *The Clock of Ages*. New York, N.Y., Cambridge University Press.

Michener, J. (1994). *Recessional*. New York, N.Y., Random House.

Moir, A. and Jessel, D. (1991). *Brain Sex*. New York, N.Y., Carol Publishing Group.

Morgan, B. and Morgan, R. (1987). *Brainfood*. Tucson, Ariz., The Body Press.

Moyers, B. (1993). *Healing and The Mind*. New York, N.Y., Doubleday.

National Geographic Society. (1998). *Incredible Voyage: Exploring the Human Body*. Washington, D.C.

Nuland, S. (1997). *The Wisdom of the Body*. New York, N.Y. Knopf.

Ornstein, R. (1997). *The Right Mind*. New York, N.Y., Harcourt Brace.

Pierpaoli, W., Regelson, W. and Colman, C. (1995). *The Melatonin Miracle*. New York, N.Y., Simon and Schuster.

Purves, D. et al. (1997) *Neuroscience*. Sunderland, Mass. Sinauer.

Posner, M., and Raichle, M (1994). *Images of Mind*. New York, N.Y., Freeman.

Rayner, C. (1990). *Atlas of the Body and Mind*. Chicago, Ill., Rand McNally.

Restak, R. (1997). *Older and Wiser*. New York, N.Y. Simon Schuster.

Restak, R. (1994). *Receptors*. New York, N.Y., Bantam Books.

Restak. R. (1991). *The Brain Has A Mind of Its Own*. New York, N.Y., Harmony Books.

Restak, R. (1988). *The Mind*. New York, N.Y., Bantam Books.

Reiter, R. and Robinson, J. (1995). *Melatonin*. New York, N.Y., Bantam Books.

Ricklefs, R. and Finch, C. (1995). *Aging, A Natural History*. New York, N.Y., Scientific American Library.

Rodgers, J. (1992). *Psychosurgery*. New York, N.Y., HarperCollins.

Stein, D., Brailowsky, S. and Will, B. (1996) *Brain Repair*. New York, N.Y., Oxford University Press.

Sylvia, C. and Nowak, W. (1997). *A Change of Heart*. New York, N.Y., Little, Brown.

Sylwester, R. (1995). *Celebration of Neurons*. Alexandria, Va., ASCD.

Time-Life. (1994). *Repair and Renewal*. Alexandria, Va., Time-Life Books.

Ulatowska, H. (1985). *The Aging Brain, Communication in the Elderly*. San Diego, Calif., College-Hill Press.

Vaughn, C. (1996). *How Life Begins*. New York, N.Y. Doubleday.

Weiss, S. and Feinberg, A. (1995). *Live Longer, Live Better*. Pleasantville, N.Y., Readers Digest Association.

Williams, M. (1995). *Complete Guide to Aging and Health*. New York, N.Y., Harmony Books.